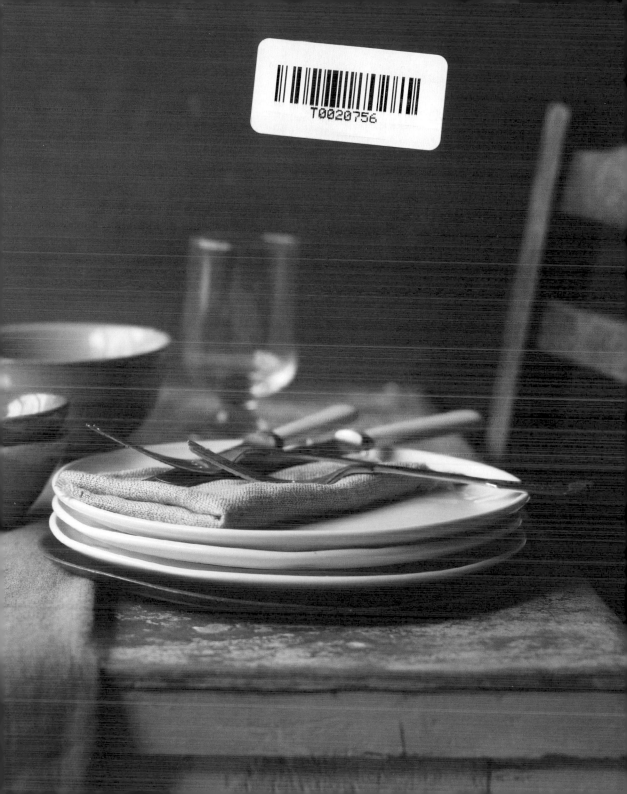

the GUILT-FREE kitchen

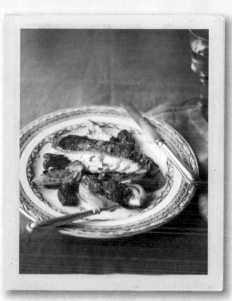

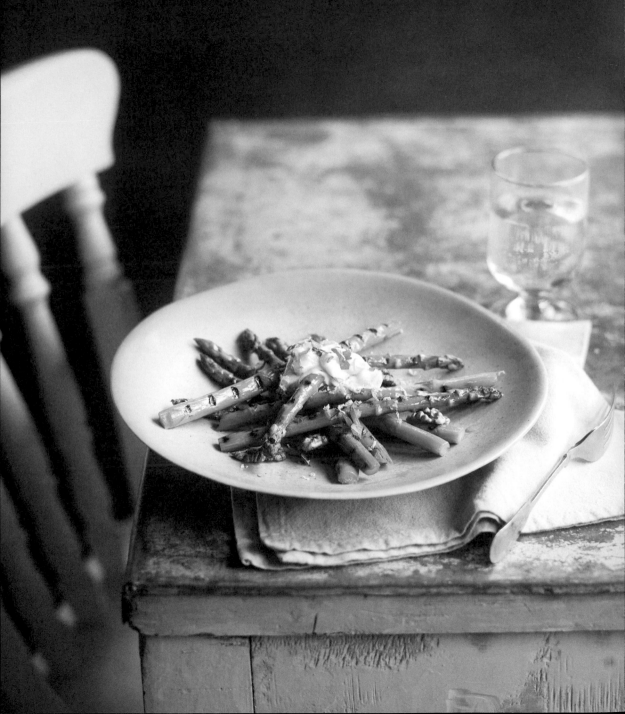

the GUILT-FREE kitchen

INDULGENT RECIPES WITHOUT REFINED SUGAR, WHEAT OR DAIRY

JORDAN & JESSICA BOURKE

Photography by KATE WHITAKER

RYLAND PETERS & SMALL

LONDON • NEW YORK

Senior Designer Megan Smith
Commissioning Editor Céline Hughes
Production Manager Gordana Simakovic
Art Director Leslie Harrington
Editorial Director Julia Charles
Publisher Cindy Richards

Food Stylist Jordan Bourke
Prop Stylist Liz Belton
Indexer Hilary Bird

First published in 2012 and reissued
in 2019 as *The Guilt-Free Gourmet*.
This revised edition published in 2022
by Ryland Peters & Small
20–21 Jockey's Fields,
London WC1R 4BW
and
341 E 116th Street, New York, 10029
www.rylandpeters.com

10 9 8 7 6 5 4 3 2 1

ISBN: 978-1-78879-443-5

Printed and bound in China

A CIP record for this book is available
from the British Library.
US Library of Congress Cataloging-in-
Publication Data has been applied for.

Notes

• Both British (Metric) and American
(Imperial plus US cups) measurements
are included in these recipes for your
convenience, however it is important
to work with one set of measurements
and not alternte between the two
within a recipe.
• All spoon measurements are level,
unless otherwise specified.
• Ovens should be preheated to the
specified temperature. Recipes in this
book were tested using a regular oven.
If using a fan-assisted/convection oven,
follow the manufacturer's instructions
for adjusting temperatures.
• All eggs are medium (UK) or large
(US), unless otherwise specified. It is
recommended that free-range, organic
eggs be used whenever possible.
Recipes containing raw or partially
cooked egg, or raw fish or shellfish,
should not be served to the very
young, very old, anyone with a
compromised immune system or
pregnant women.

• When a recipe calls for the grated zest
of citrus fruit, buy unwaxed fruit and
wash well before use. If you can only find
treated fruit, scrub well in warm soapy
water and rinse before using.
• This is not an allergy cookbook as the
recipes contain nuts and eggs as well as
other known allergens. Allergy sufferers
should carefully read the label of any
product they buy for a recipe in this
book, to ensure it is free of whatever
ingredient they are allergic to.
• While we use alternatives to wheat in
this cookbook, unfortunately we cannot
guarantee all recipes are gluten free,
as we use a number of ingredients that
contain gluten, but not wheat. If you are
coeliac, please substitute for gluten-free
alternatives. Products such as oats, soy
sauce, sausages, etc., are available free
of gluten if required.
• Products such as mirin, rice milk,
gochujang, dark chocolate, etc., are
available free of cane sugar if required.

Disclaimer

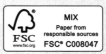

contents

the guilt-free gourmet

'You are what you eat' seems like such an obvious statement, so why then is it so hard to eat well and satisfy our cravings in a healthy way? This cookbook is for all those people who are tired of being told to eat more fruit and vegetables and reduce their intake of refined and processed foods, but who are rarely given any recipes or advice on how to put those guidelines into practice in a way that doesn't compromise on the flavour and enjoyment of our food. This is also for the growing number of people who are suffering from intolerances to certain food groups, particularly wheat and dairy. While there is nothing wrong with either food group, if you find yourself no longer able to tolerate them, this book will give you some great alternative options. For those with severe allergies, we do use nuts, eggs and other known allergen products, so do please adjust any of the recipes to suit your own needs.

This cookbook is not about diet, weight loss or denial; it is simply showing you the various ways you can use alternative ingredients to achieve the same decadent results as the original. If you are looking for a low calorie diet book, look away now, our recipes are abundant, delicious and in some cases indulgent, so the old adage of 'everything in moderation' still holds true here.

Ask yourself how many times you have seen a friend go for a wheat-free sandwich, sugar-free snack bar or dairy-free soy latte? The demand for delicious alternatives is already huge and ever increasing. With this in mind we set about combining our expertise as a chef and nutritional therapist to show you the amazing range of dishes you can cook for yourself at home.

While you are whipping up one of the dishes, you can also read the accompanying nutritional fact boxes which explain the health benefits of certain ingredients. The three main foods that come up time and time again with my sister's nutrition clients and my private cooking clients are refined cane sugar, processed wheat and dairy. These are the three ingredients that all of our clients have had issues with. So instead we use alternatives to achieve the same results. Things like natural maple syrup and coconut palm sugar keep things sweet, while spelt and rice flour help to keep things light and soy cream/creamer and rice milk provide the creaminess. Of course, nobody wants to trek halfway across the country to get these things, so we have made sure that most of the ingredients used are available in a good supermarket. Failing that, the furthest you will have to go is a health food store, branches of which, due to high demand, are popping up all over the place.

As a chef, taste and seasoning are of paramount importance. My sister has also learned from experience that no one, no matter how determined, will be able to stick to a diet that is overly bland or virtuous in comparison to what they are used to. For all of our clients the idea that they could eat rich desserts like chocolate brownies and ice cream that are free from cane sugar, wheat and dairy, yet still taste great, was almost impossible to believe. This is what made it so easy for them to make the change, as unlike anything else out there, it is not about denial. The improvements to their general health were also a great incentive to keep going, with a noticeable difference in a variety of areas from weight loss, better skin and fewer colds, to more restful sleep, increased energy and better concentration. For some of my sister's fertility clients, this change in their diet was also instrumental in achieving a healthy pregnancy.

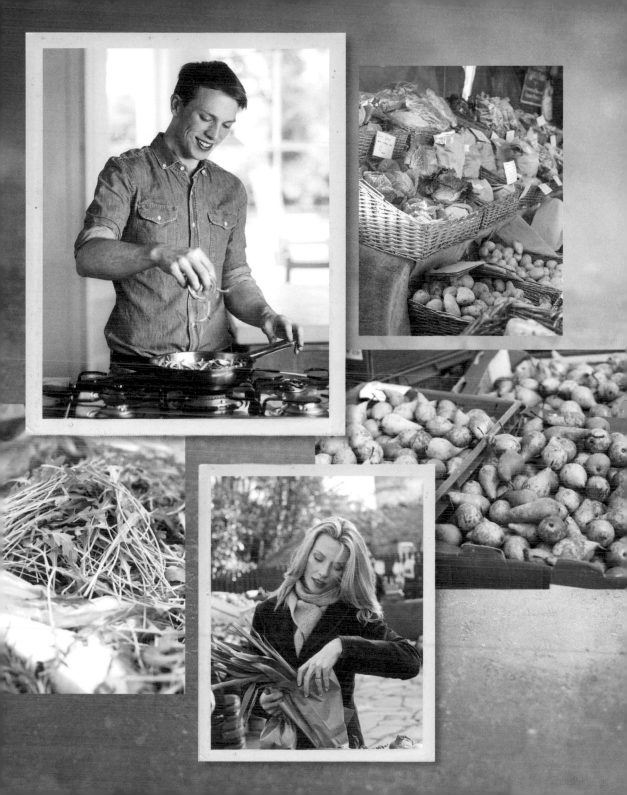

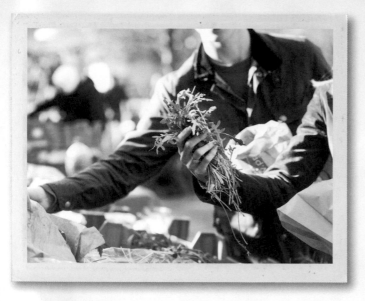

days a week, we can then afford to spend a little more money on better quality meat on the days we do choose to eat it.

Cooking relies as much on instinct and common sense as it does on following a recipe word for word. The size and water content of a vegetable can vary wildly from one to another, no two ovens are created equal which can affect cooking times dramatically, and sometimes measurements will be slightly off in the recipe: for example, if you are making a pastry on a particularly wet day, the flour will absorb some of the moisture in the air and therefore not require as much of the liquid in the recipe. So trust your instincts and taste buds, as that is how you will become a good cook. If the cake looks and feels done 10 minutes before the end of the marked cooking time, take it out. If you think your dish could take a bit more seasoning than has been specified, go for it. After all, it is you that has to eat the end result.

Of course, not everyone has a problem with cane sugar, wheat and dairy and even if they did, few of us would be willing to give up these foods for the rest of our lives. However, what everyone does have in common is the knowledge that eating too many sugary and fatty foods can have negative effects on our health. Chronic conditions such as cardiovascular disease, diabetes and obesity are now commonplace. So these recipes appeal to everyone, from those who already know they would rather cut down on these ingredients, to the general masses, who now and again want to be able to try out alternative ingredients to what they normally cook with.

As for fish and meat, I don't think I could write anything here that you haven't heard many times before. We all know how battery-farmed chickens are reared or the merits of organic meat or sustainably caught fish to our health and our environment, but not all of us can afford to take heed of this advice every day of the week, so just buy mindfully as and when you can. Paul, Mary and Stella McCartney's 'Meat Free Monday' initiative makes a lot of sense too, the idea being that if we don't eat meat seven

Points to Remember

Fats

Fat is a nutrient that is as vital to our health and diet as protein or carbohydrate is. It is just the type and quantity of fats that we are consuming that is the problem. More than 70% of the brain is composed of fat and there is a fat layer lining every single nerve and cell in the body. Without healthy fats in our diet, we would see a rapid decline in our health, so it is important to be able to distinguish between the types of fats we are consuming. Plant-based fats, such as those from nuts, seeds, avocados, coconut oil and extra virgin olive oil are high in essential fatty acids that are crucial for our health and wellbeing, from brain and nerve function, to cell growth and even weight loss. While the excessive consumption of animal-based saturated fats from meat, cheese, milk, cream etc., along with trans fats found in processed meals and certain margarines, have been found to contribute to cardiovascular disease and obesity as well as many other ailments, so the medical advice historically has been to eat this kind of fat in moderation. Given many of our most loved dishes tend to focus heavily on this kind of fat, our recipes will hopefully give you a few alternatives for the days you want to try out something else.

Sweet

We know that the quantity of processed sugar we are consuming is bad for us and extremely addictive, so what alternatives are there? Xylitol is one example. Despite its unusual name, xylitol does not belong to the class of 'artificial sweeteners' that have received bad press in recent years for their possible side-effects. It is a sweetener that the body recognizes as natural because it is present in all plant cells and is derived from tree bark. It can be used in the same way as sugar and has no impact on blood sugar levels. It also doesn't feed mouth bacteria, which means it is a better option than sugar for dental health.

Coconut palm sugar, agave, maple, date and rice syrups are some other alternatives we use in this book. However, all sugars even the so-called 'healthy' alternatives, are assimilated in the body in the same way as regular cane sugar. So they must still be eaten in moderation. The good news is wherever there is sugar in nature, for example dried and fresh fruit, there is also fibre, which slows down the rate at which sugar is absorbed into our blood, so you don't get the blood sugar peaks that you would with sugar on its own.

Wheat

Refined wheat flour has received a lot of bad press in recent years, as more and more people find themselves reacting badly to it. It seems the problem stems from the products we are eating that are made from overly refined wheat flour, such as the mass-produced bread found in supermarkets. These loaves use wheat that has been stripped of its nutrients and cultivated for high yield and consistent baking performance and plied with additives and chemicals to achieve perfect-looking bread that is permanently soft. Home bakers and artisan bakeries on the other hand, rely only on three ingredients to make their bread – flour, water and yeast – so it is probably no surprise that many of our clients have found they don't react as badly to bread made in this way, even though it still contains wheat.

As intolerances and allergies have developed, so too has the demand for recipes using more nutritious, reduced-wheat alternatives. Spelt flour (an ancient grain popular for its very similar profile to wheat, but with less gluten and a higher nutrient content) and entirely wheat-free flours like rice and gram are now increasingly in demand and it is easy to see why. In this book all of our recipes offer alternatives to wheat flour that achieve the same result.

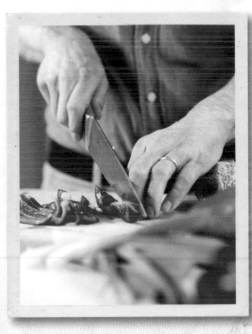

brunch

The ultimate in laidback weekend indulgence, brunch is all about taking your time, chilling out with family and friends and enjoying simple yet delicious food. Here is a selection of great brunch dishes that take no time at all to whip up, from smoothies and granola to pancakes and bread… and all guilt free!

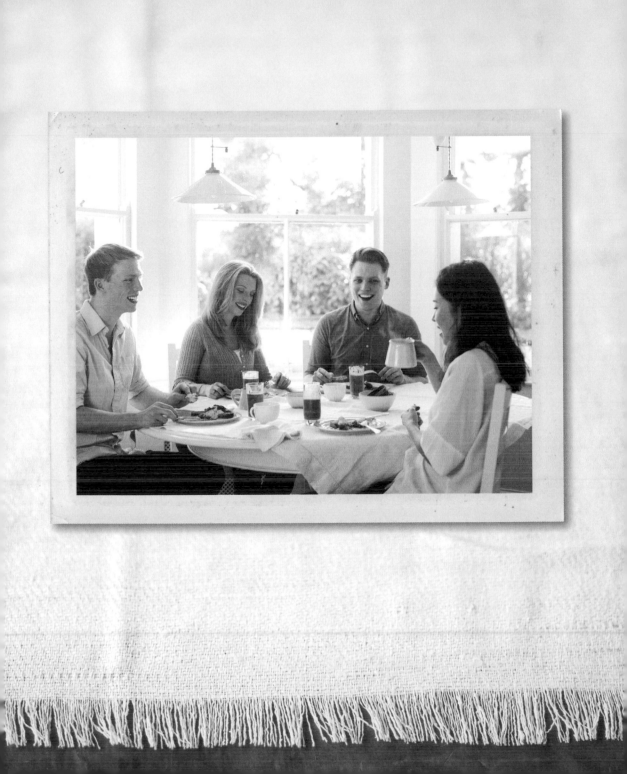

Smoothies really are the perfect way to incorporate superfoods into your diet. These three recipes will introduce you to lucuma, maca and goji berries, which you can easily find in health stores and some good supermarkets. Packed with antioxidants, vitamins and minerals, they provide your body with a natural immune and stamina booster.

super smoothies

mango lucuma lassi

3 ripe mangoes, pitted and peeled
220 ml/1 scant cup rice milk
450 g/15 oz. soy yogurt
2 tablespoons agave or maple syrup
grated zest and juice of 1 lime
a pinch of sea salt
1 tablespoon lucuma
good pinch of ground cardamom, plus extra to dust

Serves 3–4

In a blender, blitz together all the ingredients until smooth, keeping aside a little lime zest. Pour into tall glasses and serve with a pinch of cardamom and lime zest on top.

frozen banana, cocoa & maca smoothie

4 very ripe bananas, peeled, chopped and frozen in a resealable bag
400 ml/1⅔ cups rice milk
1 teaspoon ground cinnamon
1 teaspoon maca powder
2 teaspoons unsweetened cocoa powder

Serves 3–4

In a blender, put a few chunks of banana with enough rice milk to cover them. Blitz until smooth, then keep adding the bananas and rice milk until well blended. Add the remaining ingredients and blitz until smooth. Pour into tall glasses and serve immediately.

raspberry, blueberry & goji berry smoothie

400 g/14 oz. frozen raspberries and blueberries
2 tablespoons goji berries
200 ml/6½ oz. soy yogurt
400 ml/1⅔ cups rice milk
2 teaspoons agave syrup

Serves 3–4

In a blender, blitz together all the ingredients until smooth. Pour into tall glasses and serve immediately.

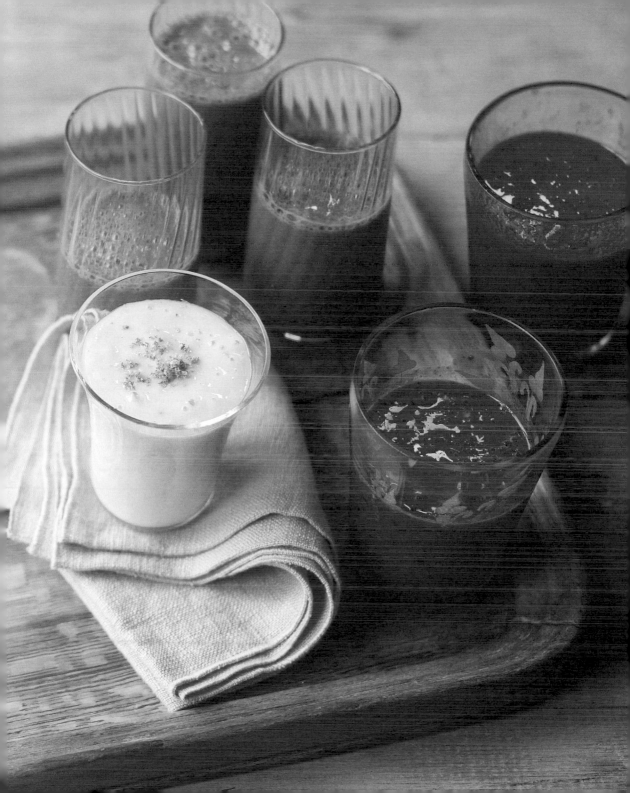

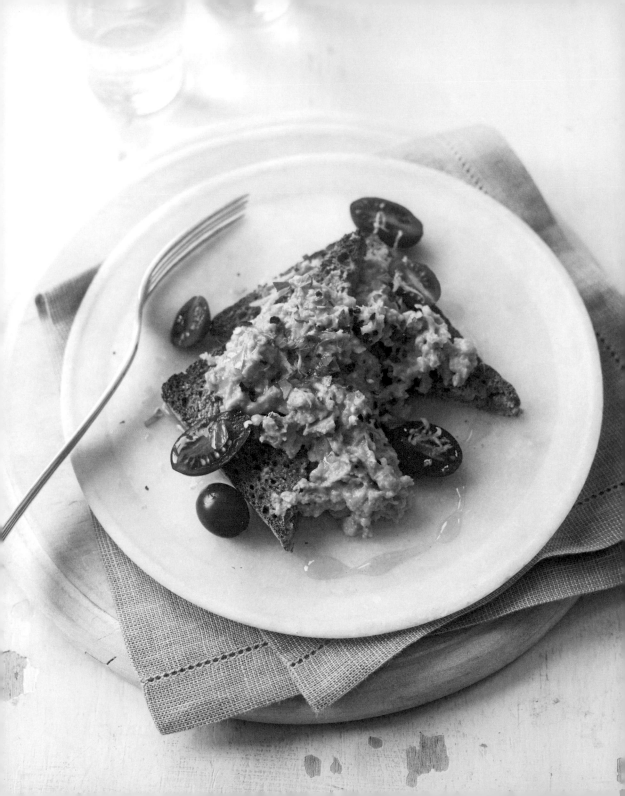

When I lived in New York, I became obsessed with the avocado toast served at the wonderful Café Gitane in SoHo. Back in London though, I had no choice but to make my own version of it. For a glorious breakfast, I serve it on the Village Bakery brand of rye bread. I think it's hands down the best rye bread in the UK — they don't use any white flour yet still manage to get a good rise, so unlike many other rye breads it is not like concrete. I've thrown some cherry tomatoes into this dish as well but you must use the most vibrant red tomatoes you can find.

new york avocado toast

2 avocados
grated zest of 1 lemon,
  plus juice of ½ lemon
1 tablespoon freshly
  chopped parsley
extra virgin olive oil
sea salt

7 cherry tomatoes
2 slices rye or wheat-free
  bread
sprinkling of dried chilli
  /red pepper flakes

Serves 2

Cut the avocados in half, remove the stones and scoop the flesh into a bowl. Mash it up with a fork, leaving some chunks for texture. Season with half the lemon zest and juice, the parsley, some oil and a pinch of salt. Taste and adjust if necessary.

Halve the tomatoes and season with the remaining lemon zest and juice, some oil and a pinch of salt.

Put the bread on to toast. Cut the toast diagonally in half and divide between 2 plates. Drizzle with olive oil and a very small pinch of salt, pile the avocado on top, sprinkle with the chilli/pepper flakes and serve with the tomatoes.

Guilt-free because...

Parsley is such a common kitchen herb that it's easy to forget just how nutritious it is

It contains high levels of 'volatile oils' such as myristicin, limonene, eugenol and alpha-thujene that are known to be cancer-protective. These volatile oils have been shown to inhibit tumour formation, particularly on the lungs. Myristicin helps activate an enzyme in the body called Glutathione S-transferase. Without this enzyme we would not be able to attach Glutathione to health-damaging oxidized molecules in order to 'escort' them out of the body.

Parsley is a great source of folate so should be consumed regularly by women of child-bearing age to help prevent the occurrence of spina bifida during early pregnancy.

eggs on rye with spinach & roasted tomatoes

4 tomatoes – as ripe and
  red as you can find –
  halved
sea salt and freshly
  ground black pepper
coconut palm sugar
  (available in health
  stores)
extra virgin olive oil
4 eggs
100 ml/6 tablespoons soy
  cream/creamer
150 g/5 oz. spinach leaves
4 slices rye, spelt or
  wheat-free bread of
  your choice

Serves 4

Preheat the oven to 180°C (350°F) Gas 4.

Place the tomato halves on a baking sheet and season well with salt, pepper and coconut sugar in equal quantities. Drizzle with just a little olive oil. Bake in the preheated oven for 30 minutes, then lower the temperature to 150°C (300°F) Gas 2 and bake for another 30 minutes until the tomatoes have dried up a little and caramelized on top.

Whisk together the eggs and cream in a bowl and season with a generous pinch of salt and pepper.

Heat a saucepan over high heat, add the spinach and sprinkle over a few drops of water. Stir until the spinach has completely wilted, then drain off any excess water and season with olive oil.

Put the bread on to toast. While that is happening, over medium heat add the egg mixture to the spinach in the pan. Using a spatula, continuously move the spinach and egg mixture around as they cook. Just before you think it is ready, when it still seems a little too wet, turn off the heat.

Cut the toast diagonally in half and divide between 4 plates. Drizzle with olive oil and a very small pinch of salt, pile the egg and spinach mixture on top and arrange the tomatoes on the side. Finish off with another drizzle of olive oil and a little pepper.

There is no better way to start a weekend than with eggs on toast. Many people find that commercially produced loaves of refined and processed bread don't agree with them. Rye and spelt are a great alternative, as they have much less gluten and chemicals are less often used in their production.

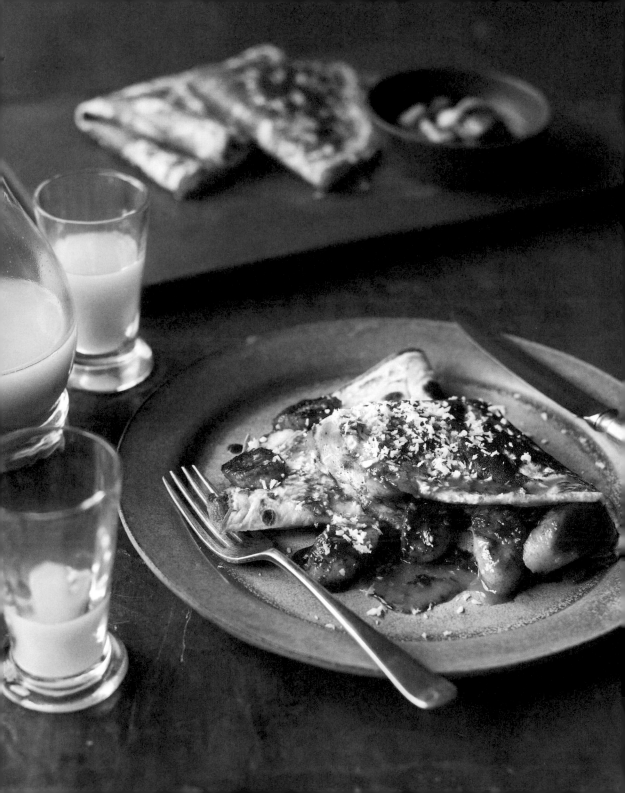

Much as I love a stack of American-style pancakes, I still prefer the French-style thin and lacy crêpe. It is just as easy to make delicious wheat-free versions, or if you can tolerate a little wheat but want a healthier option, spelt flour is better for you and has a higher mineral and vitamin content than ordinary flour. People with mild wheat intolerances generally find they can tolerate spelt with no side effects.

pancakes with fried bananas

sunflower oil, to fry

Spelt or Wheat-free
Pancakes
100 g/¾ cup fine-grind spelt flour OR 100 g/¾ cup gluten-free multi-purpose flour OR to make your own gluten-free blend, mix 50 g/6 tablespoons rice flour, 30 g/¼ cup tapioca flour, and 3 tablespoons gram flour
½ teaspoon baking powder
pinch of sea salt
2 eggs
200 ml/¾ cup rice milk

Fried Bananas
2 bananas
juice of 1 orange
2 teaspoons agave syrup
1 teaspoon ground cinnamon
1 teaspoon desiccated coconut, plus extra to serve

20–22-cm/8–10-inch non-stick frying pan

Makes about 5

To make either the spelt or wheat-free pancakes, sift the flour, baking powder and salt into a large mixing bowl and make a well in the middle.

In a separate bowl, whisk together the eggs and milk. Gradually pour into the well in the flour mixture, mixing all the time until you get a smooth batter. Allow the batter to rest for at least 30 minutes. You can also make it the night before if you are very organized.

When ready, heat a little oil in the non-stick frying pan until hot. Stir the batter and pour a small ladleful into the pan, swirling so that the mixture spreads to the edges. Cook until the top of the pancake starts to bubble – less than 1 minute – then flip it over

and cook until golden. Repeat until all the batter has been used up, wrapping the pancakes in parchment paper and keeping warm in a low oven.

To make the fried bananas, heat a little oil in a frying pan over high heat. Slice the bananas and add to the hot pan. Fry until golden, then flip over and fry another minute or so. Add the orange juice and agave syrup and dust the cinnamon and desiccated coconut over the top. Let the liquid bubble away for 30 seconds, then remove from the heat and transfer to a bowl.

Add some of the fried bananas to each pancake and fold it over into a parcel. Sprinkle over a little more coconut and enjoy immediately.

Guilt-free because…

Banana is widely known for its potential to reduce hypertension due to the high amounts of potassium it contains, coupled with negligible sodium levels. It is not only the potassium but also the fibre that contributes to the cardio-protective effect.

This is the fastest bread to make and with the minimum of fuss as you don't have to knead it or allow it to rise. It's perfect on a Sunday morning slathered with some butter and jam. There are excellent quality dairy-free butters and sugar-free jams available these days, so you really can indulge without the guilt.

spelt bread

475 g/3⅔ cups wholegrain spelt flour (this contains a small amount of gluten, so it is not suitable for coeliacs)
1 teaspoon baking powder
1 teaspoon bicarbonate of/baking soda
1 teaspoon sea salt

50 g/⅓ cup raisins
150 g/1 cup mixed seeds (eg. sunflower, pumpkin, flaxseed etc.)
1 tablespoon blackstrap molasses
550 ml/2⅓ cups tepid water

20-cm/8-inch loaf pan, greased and lined with parchment paper

Makes 1 loaf

Preheat the oven to 180°C (350°F) Gas 4.

Mix all the dry ingredients together in a large mixing bowl.

Mix together the molasses and tepid water until well blended. Add to the dry ingredients and mix together until combined.

Pour into the prepared loaf pan and bake in the preheated oven for 1 hour or until well risen.

Allow to cool, then enjoy in thick slices with dairy-free butter, sugar-free jam and a cup of tea.

Guilt-free because...

Spelt is technically an ancient form of wheat, but it is easier to digest than standard wheat, higher in protein and the B-complex vitamins, while also having a lower gluten content. Gluten is the protein contained in numerous grains that can cause severe reactions in sensitive individuals, namely coeliacs. While spelt is not a safe grain for coeliacs to consume, for the rest of us it's a good alternative to standard wheat, as many people who have a wheat intolerance find they fare better with spelt bread.

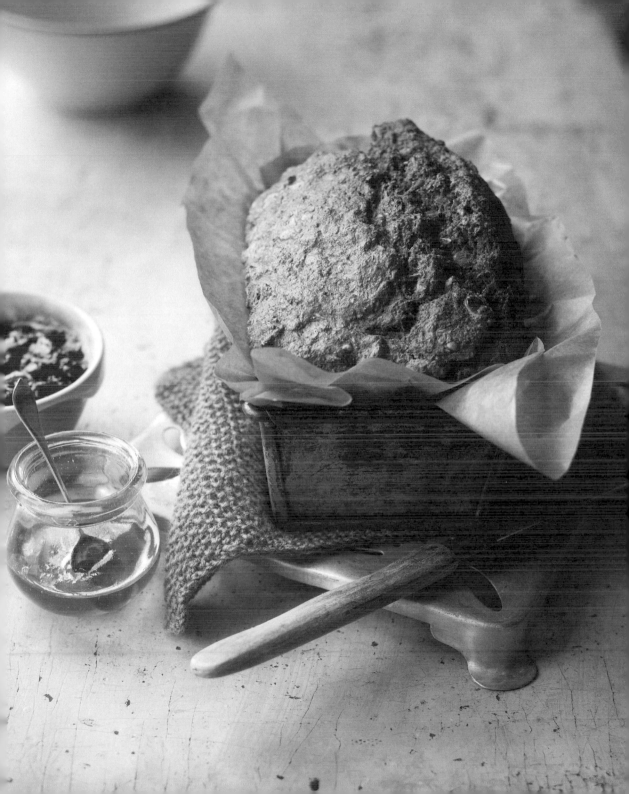

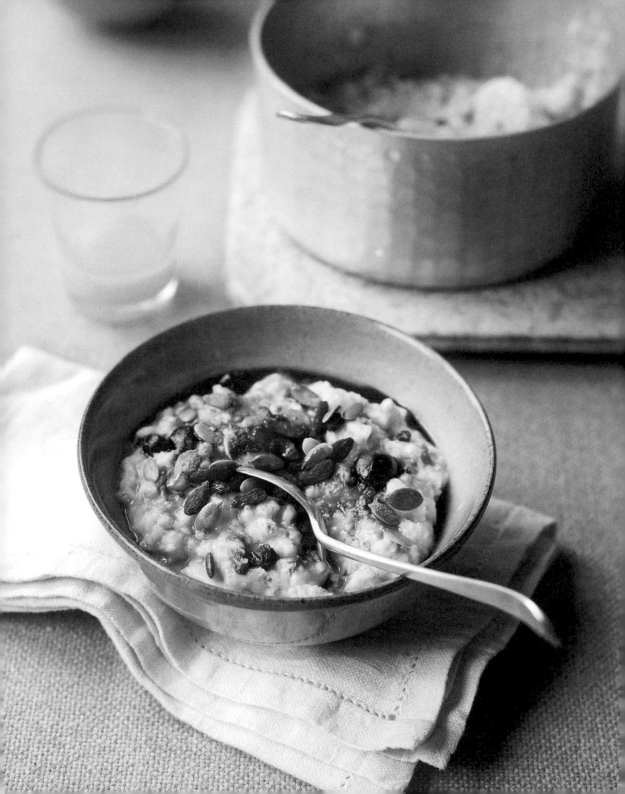

For the majority of the year, I survive on porridge to get me through the mornings, moving onto bircher muesli when it is warm enough to tolerate a cold breakfast. Porridge is nourishing, sustaining and crucially, not rammed full of refined white sugar and processed sodium chloride salt, like the majority of breakfast cereals out there. So you won't have any energy crashes at 11:30 when your body comes down off the sugar. Below are suggested ingredients you can use.

porridge

130 g/1 cup jumbo rolled oats

rice milk (or soy or nut milk)

fresh fruit, eg. bananas, berries (fresh or frozen), apples, pears, persimmons, cherries

dried fruit, eg. raisins, unsulphured apricots, dates, mango etc.

spices, eg. ground ginger, cinnamon, nutmeg

sweeteners, eg. agave syrup, pure maple syrup, rice syrup, date syrup, coconut palm sugar

(remember that if you have used a fair amount of fresh and dried fruit, the porridge will be naturally sweet and may not need anything else)

nuts and seeds, eg. almonds, cashews, pecans, macadamia nuts sunflower seeds, hemp seeds, pumpkin seeds, flaxseeds etc.

superfoods, eg. goji berries, maca powder, lucuma powder

Serves 2

Put the oats in a saucepan and cover with half water and half rice milk. Cook gently over low–medium heat, stirring more and more frequently as they begin to thicken. Oats absorb a huge amount of liquid, so they become thick and gloopy very quickly. Some people love it at this consistency, but if, like me, you prefer your porridge a little more runny, then just keep adding more rice milk and water until you reach the desired consistency. Only add a little at a time though, so you don't overdo it. When it is ready, turn it right down to the lowest heat.

Now add whatever selection of ingredients you like the sound of. My personal favourite is banana, raisins, ground cinnamon, pumpkin seeds, goji berries and the tiniest drop of pure maple syrup. It is insanely good and brightens up even the gloomiest of Monday mornings. I also love adding frozen blueberries, which defrost in the hot porridge leaving lovely cool pockets of sweetness. You can go wild with all the possibilities and the positive effect that the warm porridge will have on your outlook for the day, waistline and (ahem) 'regularity' are all added bonuses!

Guilt-free because…

Porridge can be as healthy or as unhealthy as you like. While many of us are inclined to add milk, cream and sugar, porridge is the perfect vessel for all manner of superfood ingredients. Goji berries, for example, are a tangy red fruit harvested from the Himalayas and the only known fruit to contain all 8 essential amino acids. They are high in vitamin C and contain 15 times more iron than spinach, which ensures efficient absorption of this crucial mineral.

Granola is absolutely one of the simplest things you can make in a kitchen, plus it costs half the price and tastes infinitely better than the storebought stuff... in my opinion!

granola

125 ml/½ cup pure maple syrup

125 ml/½ cup agave syrup

200 ml/¾ cup flavourless oil, eg. sunflower or grapeseed

2 teaspoons ground cinnamon

800 g/6½ cups jumbo oats

200 g/1½ cups mixed nuts, and seeds eg. pecans, hazelnuts, cashews and pumpkin seeds

150 g/1 cup raisins

150 g/1 cup chopped unsulphured dried apricots

Serves 10–12

Preheat the oven to 180°C (350°F) Gas 4.

Mix together the maple and agave syrups, oil and cinnamon. In a large mixing bowl, combine the oats and oil mixture until all the oats are evenly coated.

Spread the oats out on 2 baking sheets and bake in the preheated oven for about 20–30 minutes until they turn a lovely golden brown. Give them a stir once or twice during cooking to make sure they are all evenly cooked. If it looks like they might be burning, turn the oven temperature down slightly and stir them again.

While the oats are in the oven, you can also roast the mixed nuts and seeds for 10–15 minutes or until they go a shade darker and their flavours are released.

Let the oats and nuts cool down, then mix together with the raisins and apricots. If you feel like you want more cinnamon feel free to add more at this stage.

A word to the wise: resist the temptation to mix all the ingredients together and bake as one. The reason being that the dried fruit burns alarmingly quickly and ruins the granola, as it takes on a bitter taste. The nuts also cook faster than the oats, so it is better to cook them separately.

I am not sure whether it has something to do with the fact that I am Irish, but oats have always been a mainstay in my breakfast choices. Whether lightly toasted in a granola, cooked on the hob for porridge or soaked and served with yogurt, nuts and fruit like this bircher muesli, they always seem to do the trick. Served at room temperature, bircher muesli is the perfect choice for those spring and summer mornings when you are in less need of warming porridge.

bircher muesli

300 g/2½ cups jumbo oats

150 g/1 cup mixed seeds, eg. pumpkin, sunflower, flaxseed etc.

2 apples, cored and grated

175 ml/⅔ cup rice milk

175 ml/⅔ cup apple or orange juice

100 g/⅔ cup raisins

50 g/⅓ cup dried cranberries

80 ml/⅓ cup pure maple or agave syrup

1–2 teaspoons ground cinnamon

400 ml/1¾ cups soy yogurt

Serves 4

In a large bowl, mix together all the ingredients apart from the yogurt. Allow to soak for at least 1 hour until the oats have softened, or overnight. The mixture will thicken up considerably once soaked.

When ready to eat, taste and add more maple or agave syrup and cinnamon if required. Serve it up in with as much yogurt as you like alongside it. You can mix it altogether for a looser bircher or you can dip into it as you please for a thicker consistency.

The wonderful thing about bircher muesli is that you can add whichever nuts, seeds and fruit you like, so you can really make it your own.

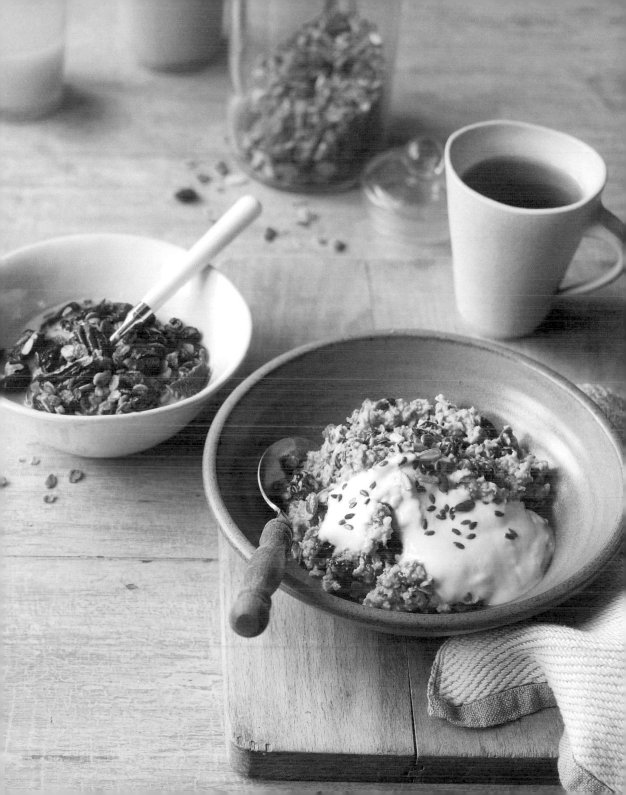

sharing plates

For me, the most enjoyable way of eating is to have family and friends gathered around a table full of food, all diving in and helping themselves as and when they please. With delicious sharing plates like frittata, meatballs, falafel and fritters you will have plenty to choose from for exactly this kind of laidback affair.

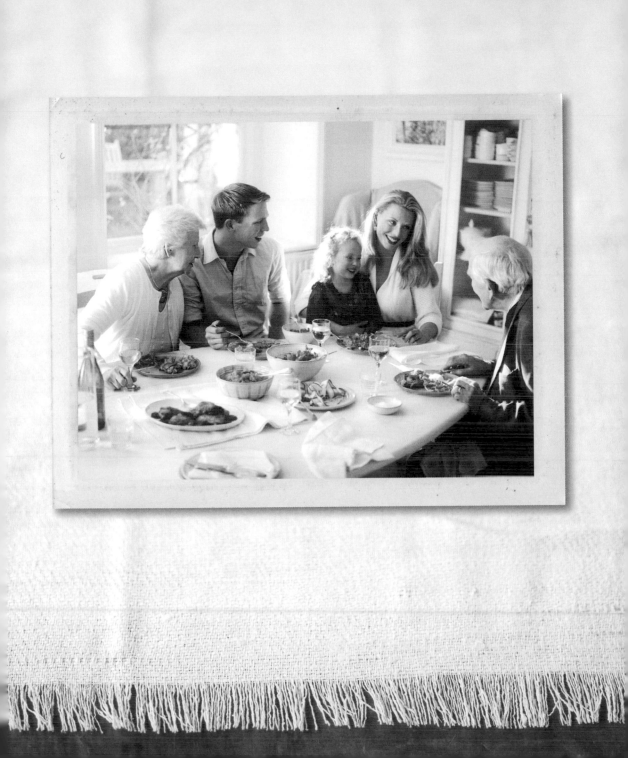

Eggs can be thrown together in all manner of ways and with wonderful results. I often make a frittata with whatever vegetables I happen to have, but this is my favourite, the vibrant emerald green cavolo nero, orange sweet potato and red tomato vying for attention. Substitute spinach if you can't find cavolo nero.

sweet potato, cavolo nero & plum tomato frittata with basil oil

1 sweet potato
extra virgin olive oil
sea salt and freshly
   ground black pepper
dried chilli/hot red
   pepper flakes
2 red onions, sliced
handful of ripe baby
   plum tomatoes
2 tablespoons good
   balsamic vinegar
bunch of cavolo nero
   leaves
10–12 eggs, depending on
   the size of your pan
small bunch of fresh basil
1 garlic clove

20–25-cm/8–10-inch
   ovenproof frying pan
   or quiche dish

Serves 8–10

Preheat the oven to 180°C (350°F) Gas 4.

Cut the potato in half lengthways and then into thin wedges. Toss in a roasting pan with 2 tablespoons olive oil and a little salt, pepper and dried chilli/red pepper flakes. Roast in the preheated oven until just browned and starting to blister.

About 15 minutes before the sweet potato is done, toss the red onions and tomatoes on a baking sheet with a few tablespoons of oil, the vinegar and a sprinkling of salt and place in the oven. The skins of the tomatoes should have just popped open and the red onions begun to caramelize when the sweet potato is ready to take out. Leave the oven on for the frittata.

Remove the cavolo nero leaves from their stalks and blanch in salted boiling water for about 2 minutes. Remove and refresh with cold water.

Crack the eggs into a bowl, whisk and season well.

Place the sweet potato, cavolo nero, tomatoes and onion (reserving some for on top) in the ovenproof frying pan or a quiche dish. Pour the beaten eggs over the top and finish with the reserved vegetables on top so that you can see their colour.

Cook in the oven for 25 minutes or until the frittata has puffed up and the top is just firm to the touch.

In the meantime, finely chop the basil and garlic and combine with 6 tablespoons olive oil to make a loose basil oil.

Allow the frittata to cool a little, then drizzle the basil oil over it and serve with a light mixed leaf salad.

Guilt-free because…

Cavolo nero, also known as **Tuscan kale,** is a nutrient powerhouse. It is rich in plant chemicals called polyphenolic flavonoids such as lutein, beta-carotene and zeaxanthin, which are known to support the health of the eyes – they may help to prevent macular degeneration. 100 g/3½ oz. provides 5 times the recommended daily allowance of vitamin A and 7 times that of vitamin K, which are needed for healthy skin and bones.

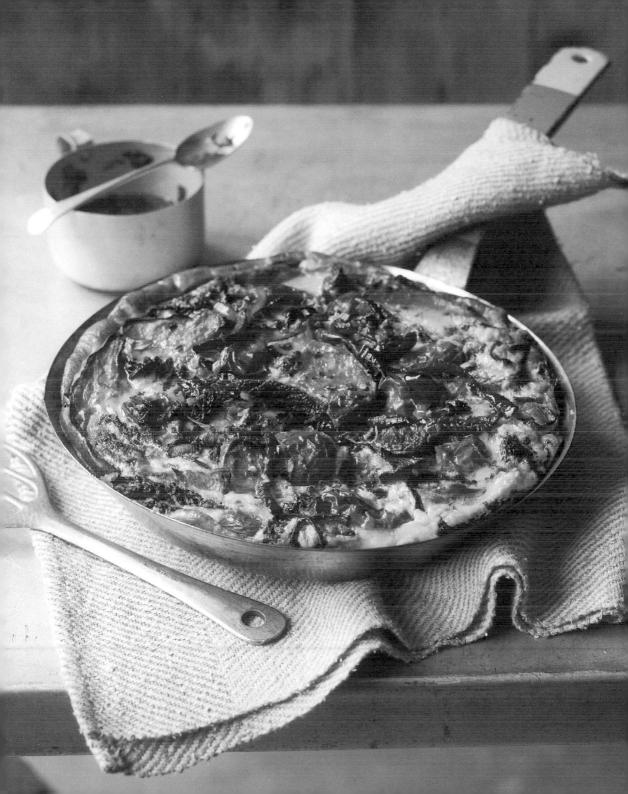

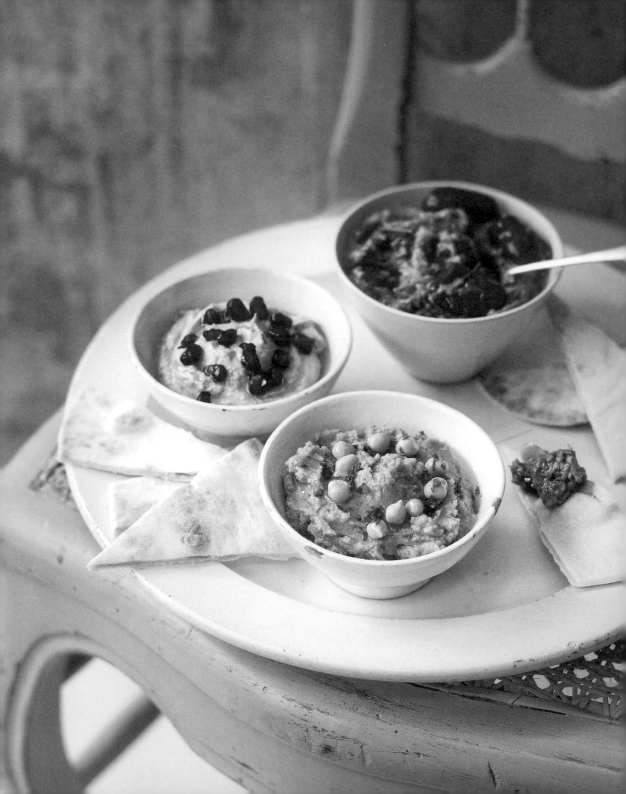

sweet potato hummus

1 large sweet potato,
   baked until very tender
400-g/14-oz. can
   chickpeas
2 garlic cloves, peeled
100 ml/6 tablespoons
   tahini
½ teaspoon each cumin
   and coriander seeds,
gently toasted in a dry
   pan until fragrant
grated zest and juice of
   ½ lemon
extra virgin olive oil
sea salt
1 tablespoon freshly
   chopped parsley

Serves 8

Scoop the flesh out of the potato. Put the flesh, chickpeas (reserving a few to garnish), garlic and tahini in a food processor and blitz together until well combined. Using a pestle and mortar, pound the cumin and coriander seeds until finely ground. Add to the processor (reserving a pinch to garnish) with the lemon zest and juice, 1 teaspoon salt and about 3 tablespoons olive oil. Blitz again until really smooth. If it is still quite stiff, add more olive oil and blitz until you have a soft, smooth purée. Season to taste.

Serve in a bowl with the reserved chickpeas, spices and parsley sprinkled over the top and some olive oil drizzled over.

baba ghanoush

2 aubergines/eggplants
2 garlic cloves, peeled
4 tablespoons tahini
3 tablespoons lemon juice
½ teaspoon sea salt
generous pinch of sweet
   smoked paprika
2 tablespoons extra virgin
   olive oil
1 tablespoon
   pomegranate seeds

Serves 8

Light 2 of the rings of your gas hob/burner on the lowest setting. Pierce the flesh of the aubergines/eggplants once or twice and place directly onto the flame. Char the skin all over, turning now and again. It should be quite charred and the flesh inside very soft – it will take longer than you think. The skin will blister and tear a little, exposing the flesh. Once completely charred, sit the aubergines/eggplants on a plate and allow to cool completely. Carefully peel away all the skin. Keep any juice that comes out, as it contains a lot of flavour.

Put aubergine/eggplant flesh, garlic, tahini, lemon juice, salt, paprika and olive oil in a food processor. Blitz until smooth. You want it to taste alive and the seasoning is key to this, so don't be mean about it.

Serve in a bowl with a little more olive oil drizzled over and slightly stirred through, and the pomegranate seeds sprinkled over the top.

borlotti bean purée

250 g/1⅔ cups dried
   borlotti beans (or fresh
   ones in the summer)
400 ml/1⅔ cups extra
   virgin olive oil
2 tablespoons red wine
   vinegar
5 garlic cloves, peeled
a few sprigs fresh
   rosemary
handful of baby plum
   tomatoes
sea salt

Serves 8

If using dried beans, put in a bowl and cover with 3 times their volume of water. Allow to soak overnight.

The next day, refresh the beans with clean water and place in a large ovenproof pot. If you are using fresh beans, then you can start from this stage. Do not add any salt at this stage, as this will prevent the beans from softening. Bring almost to the boil, then cover and reduce to a gentle simmer for about 1 hour or until they're almost tender but not completely soft.

Preheat the oven to 200°C (400°F) Gas 6.

Drain most of the water, leaving about 100 ml/ ½ cup at the bottom, add the olive oil, vinegar, garlic, rosemary, tomatoes and 1 teaspoon salt. Bake in the preheated oven for 30 minutes or until the beans have become soft and soaked up some of the liquid. Remove from the oven and allow to cool. Taste and add salt and vinegar if necessary.

Pull the leaves of the rosemary off the woody stalk, discard the stalk and put the leaves back in the pot. Bash everything with a potato masher until roughly mashed up with the oil. Season to taste one last time if necessary.

butternut squash falafels with fig, chioggia beetroot & chilli oil

extra virgin olive oil
sea salt
1 chioggia beet(root),
  very thinly sliced
radicchio leaves
handful of lamb's lettuce
  or rocket/arugula
grated zest and juice of
  1 lemon
4 fresh figs
1 fresh red chilli, seeded
  and finely chopped
balsamic vinegar

Falafel
1 butternut squash,
  peeled, seeded and cut
  into chunks
1 teaspoon each cumin
  and coriander seeds,
  gently toasted in a dry
  pan until fragrant
1 teaspoon ground
  cinnamon
2 garlic cloves, peeled
3 tablespoons freshly
  chopped coriander/
  cilantro
squeeze of lemon juice
4–6 tablespoons gram
  flour

Serves 4–6

Preheat the oven to 200°C (400°F) Gas 6.

To make the falafel, toss the butternut squash with some oil and salt on a baking sheet. Roast in the preheated oven for about 30 minutes or until the squash takes on a little colour and is cooked through.

Meanwhile, using a pestle and mortar, pound the cumin and coriander seeds until finely ground. Add the cinnamon, garlic and a good pinch of salt and pound again to a paste.

When the squash is cooked, remove from the oven and allow to cool slightly. Leave the oven on.

Put the squash in a mixing bowl and mash with a fork. Transfer to a sieve/strainer to drain for a few minutes, then lightly press with a spoon to drain off any remaining water. Put back in the bowl, add the spice paste, the coriander/cilantro and lemon juice and mix together. Add the gram flour a tablespoon at a time until the mixture is still quite loose and sticky but holds its shape when scooped out. Using 2 teaspoons, spoon the mixture onto a baking sheet, shaping with your fingers to create falafel shapes.

Roast in the oven for about 15–20 minutes, until they take on a bit of colour and firm up.

When the falafels are ready, season the beet(root), radicchio and lamb's lettuce with the lemon zest and juice, some olive oil and salt.

To serve, arrange the falafel and dressed salad on individual plates or a large serving dish. Tear open the figs and drizzle a little vinegar onto their flesh and around the plate. Combine the chopped chilli with some olive oil and drizzle over. Serve immediately.

Guilt-free because…

Winter squash, like butternut squash, are rich in B vitamins and vitamin C, which will help your body to cope with stress as well as support the immune system to prevent colds and allergies.

The original chickpea falafel can be a little tricky to make, so I quite like this butternut squash variety which is really simple. You could use any kind of squash really, or sweet potato works well too.

Falafel can be eaten in so many ways, shoved into pita breads or slathered with tahini on their own. Here though, I have paired them with juicy figs, chioggia beet(root) (I love their crazy colour, but you could use any variety), some bitter radicchio leaves and spicy oil to add a bit of heat. It works very well as a starter or a main dish if you pile it all up.

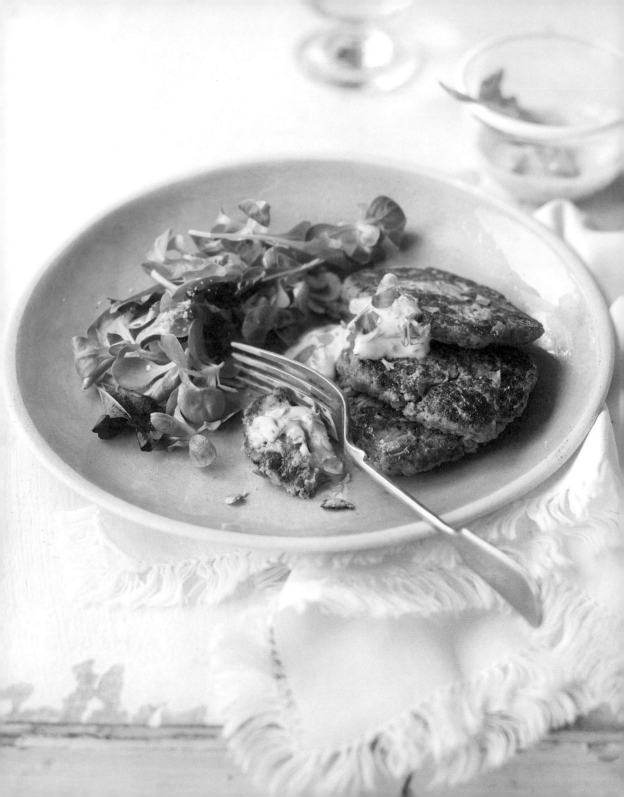

I love shopping for food in farmers' markets. The only trouble is, I often end up leaving with half the fruit and vegetable stall. These fritters were a result of one such occasion when I arrived home with far more swede/rutabaga and parsnip than I needed, so I had to invent ways of using them. I roasted some and made a soup with the rest, but my favourite use for them are these fritters, which are great.

root-vegetable fritters
with cumin & parsley yogurt

1 teaspoon cumin seeds
1 teaspoon coriander
    seeds
1 teaspoon mustard seeds
1 swede/rutabaga
2 large parsnips
extra virgin olive oil
sea salt and freshly
    ground black pepper
2 tablespoons pure maple
    syrup
½ red onion
1–2 fresh red chillies,
    seeded
½ teaspoon ground
    turmeric
handful of fresh parsley
3 eggs
2 small garlic cloves,
    peeled
1 teaspoon baking
    powder
2 teaspoons Dijon
    mustard
grated zest of 1 lemon
300 ml/1¼ cups soy
    yogurt mixed with
    1 teaspoon agave
    syrup, 1 teaspoon
    ground cumin and finely
    chopped parsley

Serves 4–6

Preheat the oven to 200°C (400°F) Gas 6.

Put the cumin, coriander and mustard seeds in a dry pan and toast for 1–2 minutes until you can smell the aromas wafting up from the pan. Pound to a powder using a pestle and mortar.

Top, tail and peel the swede/rutabaga and parsnips. Cut into small chunks and toss in a bowl with a good glug of oil, a big pinch of salt, the maple syrup and half the toasted spices. Place in a roasting pan and roast in the preheated oven for 30 minutes, or until soft and slightly caramelized. Remove from the oven and allow to cool slightly.

Spoon all the roasted ingredients, the onion, chillies, turmeric, parsley, eggs, garlic, baking powder, mustard and lemon zest into a food processor and blitz until quite smooth. Season with salt and pepper to taste.

In a large pan, heat 1 tablespoon oil over medium heat. Drop tablespoonfuls of the blitzed mixture into the pan and flatten into round shapes. Fry for a few minutes on each side or until golden. Handle gently when flipping over, as they don't firm up until fully cooked.

Serve the fritters with the sweet cumin and parsley yogurt and a green salad, if you like.

Guilt-free because…

Swede/rutabaga, typically thought of as a wartime vegetable, should not be overlooked as a root-vegetable choice. It is actually part of the 'cancer-fighting' brassica family of vegetables that includes broccoli, cauliflower and kale. These are known for their high phyto-chemical content. Eating swede/rutabaga may also be effective at increasing milk production in nursing mothers and is a high source of fibre. One serving contains over 500 mg potassium, which may help lower high blood pressure. It has also been shown to reduce the chances of cataract formation.

Without doubt my favourite way of eating is when everyone has something different and we all share! So it is no surprise that I love a good mezze, full of different textures and tastes. These mezze salads are light and fresh and balance out heavier dishes.

quinoa with carrots, hazelnuts & pomegranate

300 g/1½ cups quinoa
2 carrots, grated
60 g/½ cup hazelnuts, lightly roasted at 180°C (350°F) Gas 4 until a shade darker, then skins removed
seeds from 1 whole pomegranate
bunch of fresh parsley, chopped

10 unsulphured dried apricots, finely chopped
grated zest and juice of 1 lemon
200 ml/¾ cup extra virgin olive oil
2 tablespoons agave syrup
sea salt and freshly ground black pepper

Serves 4–6

Put the quinoa in a saucepan and cover with just under double its volume of water. Bring to the boil, then reduce the heat to low and place the lid on top. Cook for about 12 minutes until all the water has been absorbed. Turn off the heat, remove the lid and let any remaining water evaporate. Remove to a wide plate or tray and allow to cool.

Add all the remaining ingredients and 1 teaspoon salt and mix. Season to taste. Serve with more parsley sprinkled on top.

summer squash with mint & pine nuts

3 courgettes/zucchini in varying shades of green and yellow if possible
sea salt and freshly ground black pepper
small handful of fresh mint leaves

100 g/⅔ cup pine nuts, toasted until golden
grated zest and juice of ½ lemon
extra virgin olive oil

Serves 4–6

Holding a courgette/zucchini in one hand and a vegetable peeler in the other, from top to bottom peel long thin shavings of the flesh into a large bowl. Once you reach the slushy core, stop, turn the vegetable and begin peeling again. Repeat until you have worked your way around the vegetable and all you are left with is the core. Do the same with the remaining courgettes/zucchini.

Season with a good pinch of salt and pepper. Add the remaining ingredients and drizzle with olive oil.

lamb's lettuce with herbs

1–2 sprigs fresh dill
1–2 sprigs fresh tarragon
small bunch of fresh chives
grated zest and juice of 1 lemon
2 teaspoons agave syrup
1 garlic clove, crushed

1 teaspoon wholegrain mustard
3 tablespoons extra virgin olive oil
100 g/3½ oz. lamb's lettuce

Serves 4–6

Remove the dill and tarragon leaves from their stalks. Roughly chop the chives. In a small bowl, mix together the lemon zest and juice, agave syrup, garlic, mustard and oil until you have a slightly emulsified dressing. Lightly toss all the herbs and lamb's lettuce together. When ready to eat, toss with the dressing.

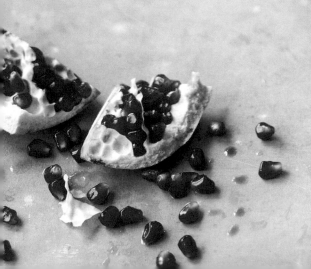

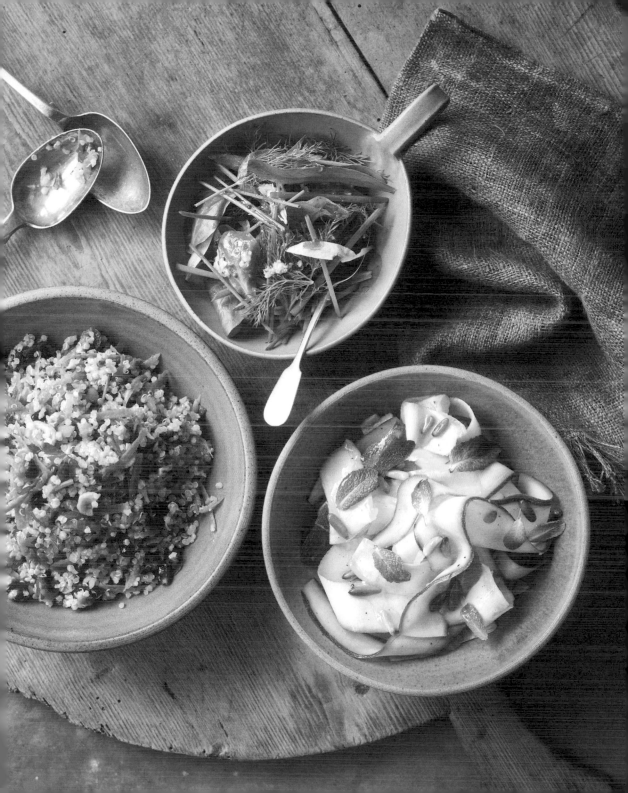

While I am delighted to see that sushi, the healthy Japanese staple, is now available in seemingly every service station and store, it's a shame that most of it is mass produced and tasteless. Sushi is actually very quick and easy to make, with the added bonus of it being up to you what you put inside it. It's ideal for a packed lunch, or plated up nicely it can be a stellar dinner party dish. This is a recipe for inside-out uramaki rolls, which look far more difficult than they actually are!

smoked mackerel sushi rolls

255 g/1¼ cups brown or white sushi rice
50 ml/3 tablespoons mirin (sweetened rice wine)
5 nori seaweed sheets
black sesame seeds
350 g/12 oz. smoked mackerel, cut into thin strips
2 spring onions/scallions, cut into thin strips
½ red (bell) pepper, cut into thick strips

To Serve
wasabi
picked Japanese sushi ginger
light soy sauce (if you have coeliac disease, use tamari soy sauce and check the label to make sure it is gluten-free)

bamboo sushi mat

Serves 4

Wash the sushi rice thoroughly under cold water and drain well. Place in a saucepan with a lid and add 550 ml/2⅓ cups water. Bring to the boil (uncovered), then reduce to the lowest heat and simmer gently until nearly all the water has been absorbed (about 20–25 minutes). Remove from the heat, place the lid on top and allow it to stand for 15 minutes to absorb the last of the water.

Spread the rice out over a clean baking sheet. Drizzle the mirin all over the rice, turning it with a spatula to help it cool down.

While it is cooling, wrap the bamboo sushi mat in clingfilm/plastic wrap, squeezing out any trapped air. This helps prevent the rice from sticking. Lay the mat lengthways in front of you. Take one nori sheet and lay it out, shiny side down, on the bamboo mat. Wet your hands and take a small handful of rice. Starting at the far end, spread and pat the rice across the nori sheet leaving a bare, ¼-cm/½-inch gap running along the edge of the sheet closest to you. You can add more rice if needed, but keep it even and no more than 1 cm/½ inch thick. If it starts sticking to your hands simply wet them again. You can also use the

back of a spoon dipped in water.

Sprinkle black sesame seeds over the rice, then flip the nori sheet over so that the rice is now facing downward with the edge free of rice still closest to you and in line with the edge of the bamboo mat. Across the middle of the nori lay 3 lines of mackerel, spring onion/scallion and red pepper.

Then, using the bamboo mat, roll the edge of the nori sheet closest to you over the filling in the middle, tucking it over firmly so the filling is enclosed. When it looks like you are about to roll the mat into the sushi roll, pull the mat back and continue to roll applying even pressure and tightening as you roll, using the mat to shape it. Once the roll has come together, carefully take it off the mat, lay the mat over it and press and smooth the roll, compressing it tightly and evening out the ends. The roll will actually be more of a rectangular shape when you have finished. With a sharp and wet knife, cut the roll in half and then each half into 3 or 4 even pieces.

Repeat this process with the remaining ingredients.

Arrange the rolls on a plate with a mound of wasabi and pickled ginger and the soy sauce in a dish on the side.

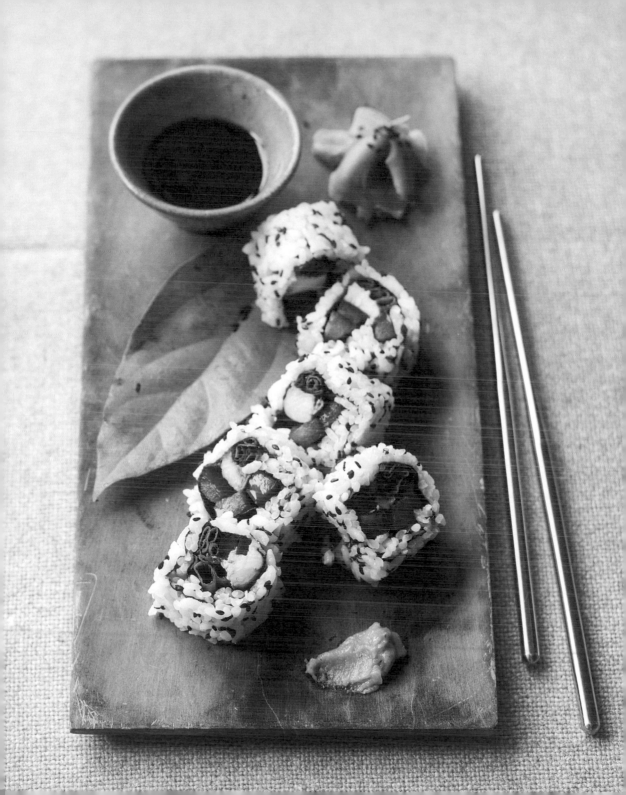

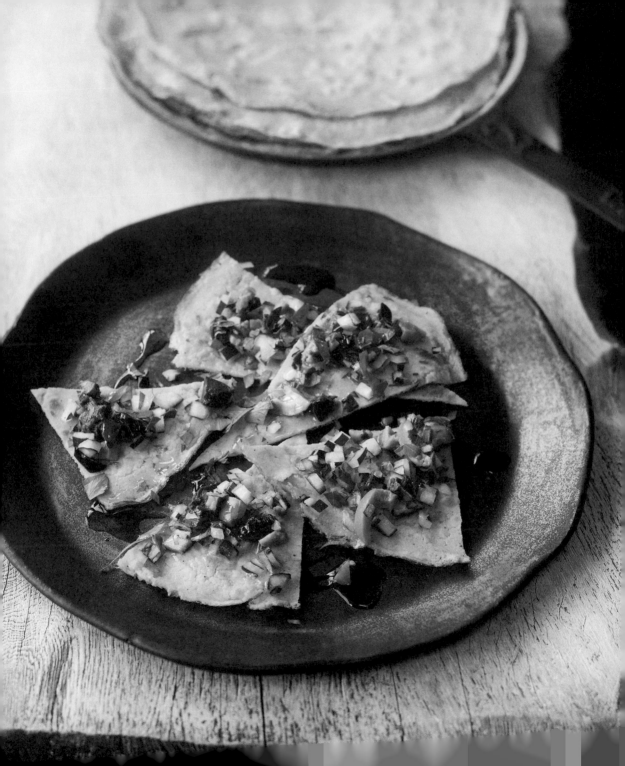

These savoury pancakes made from gram (chickpea) flour, olive oil and water hail from the Côte d'Azur in the south of France and I have loved making them ever since I discovered them there one summer, years ago. Naturally wheat and gluten free, they can be topped with just about anything you like, but the combination of chopped parsley, olives and red onion works wonderfully well.

socca

sea salt and freshly
   ground black pepper
extra virgin olive oil

Socca
150 g/1 cup plus
   2 tablespoons
   gram flour
½ teaspoon ground
   turmeric
sunflower oil

Topping
handful of pitted black
   and green olives,
   chopped into small
   chunks
2 tablespoons freshly
   chopped parsley
1 red onion, very finely
   chopped
1 lemon

20-cm/8-inch good-
   quality non-stick
   frying pan

Serves 6

To make the socca, sift the gram flour into a bowl and add ½ teaspoon salt and the turmeric. Slowly add 380 ml/ 1⅔ cups water, whisking quickly all the time until all the water has been added, breaking up any lumps of flour as you go. Add 3 tablespoons olive oil and stir.

Heat a little sunflower oil in the non-stick frying pan until hot. Pour a ladleful of the batter into the pan, swirling it so that the mixture spreads to the edges. Reduce the heat to low–medium and cook gently. It will take a good 6–8 minutes on the first side. Resist the temptation to stick your spatula underneath it until the edges have completely dried out and the middle has tiny little bubbles. At this point, take the pan and shake from side to side. The pancake should move but if it is sticking you can help it along gently with a spatula. However, if it is not

budging at all, leave it for another minute and then try again. Flip the pancake without launching it onto your kitchen ceiling, as it won't look or taste half as nice up there. Cook for a further 1 or 2 minutes. The second side does not need to be cooked for as long, as it is nice if it is still a little soft.

Repeat until all the batter has been used up, wrapping the pancakes in parchment paper and keeping warm in a low oven.

For the topping, liberally scatter the chopped olives, parsley and onion over the pancakes. Season with a good pinch of salt and pepper, a drizzle of olive oil and a squeeze of lemon juice.

Cut the pancakes into wedges, as they do in the south of France, or you can roll them up into big cigars. A little bit of hummus plopped on top works really well too, if you are so inclined.

Guilt-free because…

Red onions are high in quercetin, a bioflavonoid that is very effective at dealing with damaging free radicals. Quercetin has been described as anti-fungal, anti-bacterial and anti-inflammatory in nature. It has also been noted to inhibit the herpes zoster virus, which should bring relief to those who suffer with cold sores.

As a child in Ireland in the 1980s, I remember my mother saying it was impossible to find decent chorizo, if you could find any at all. Her solution: our Spanish au pairs smuggled chorizo back to us every time they went home to Spain. Today, luckily, authentic chorizo is easy to find. Romesco is a Spanish, nut-based sauce and a great partner to chicken and chorizo.

chicken & chorizo
with mashed squash & romesco

8 chicken thighs, skin on and bone in
extra virgin olive oil
sea salt and freshly ground black pepper
180 g/6 oz. chorizo, chopped into chunks
1 red onion, sliced
grated zest of 2 lemons
1 onion/red kuri squash, halved, seeded and cut into wedges
handful of fresh marjoram leaves

Romesco
50 g/⅓ cup almonds
30 g/3 tablespoons hazelnuts
16 ripe red plum tomatoes
1 chilli, halved and seeded
4 garlic cloves, peeled
½ teaspoon sweet smoked paprika
1–2 tablespoons red wine vinegar
4 tablespoons rye or wheat-free breadcrumbs, toasted in a little olive oil until golden

Serves 8

Preheat the oven to 200°C (400°F) Gas 6.

Coat the chicken thighs in oil, season with salt and pepper, then place in a saucepan over high heat for a few minutes, turning frequently until the skin is sealed and golden brown in colour. Transfer to a baking sheet, skin side up, and add the chorizo, onion and half the lemon zest. Roast in the preheated oven for 45 minutes or until cooked through. If they look like they are beginning to burn, turn the oven temperature down to 180°C (350°F) Gas 4 and leave them in for a little longer, or until the juices run clear when a skewer is inserted.

At the same time, on another baking sheet, toss the onion/red kuri squash with oil until well coated. Season with salt and scatter half the marjoram leaves on top. Bake in the oven for 40 minutes or until completely soft and the skin is beginning to blister.

Meanwhile, for the romesco, roast the almonds and hazelnuts on another baking sheet for 6 minutes or until they go a shade darker. Remove and allow to cool, then place the hazelnuts in a tea towel and rub off the skins.

Toss the tomatoes in oil, season with salt and the chilli and roast in the oven for about 15 minutes or until the tomato skins burst open and the chilli is soft. Using a pestle and mortar, pound the garlic, chilli, nuts and a pinch of salt until you have a chunky paste. Add the tomatoes and pound until all combined together and the skins have broken down a little. Add the paprika and vinegar. Season to taste, then add the breadcrumbs and combine together.

When the squash is cooked through, remove from the oven and place in a bowl. Season with a good pinch of salt, the remaining marjoram (reserving some for serving), the remaining lemon zest and a few glugs of oil. Mash until combined. With something like onion/red kuri squash, it really absorbs flavour and seasoning, so taste it and trust your judgment. If it needs more of anything, throw it in.

When the chicken is cooked and ready to go, scoop some of the mash onto a plate and nestle the chicken in on top, with some of the juices and chorizo scattered around. Finish with a good tablespoonful of the romesco and the reserved marjoram on top.

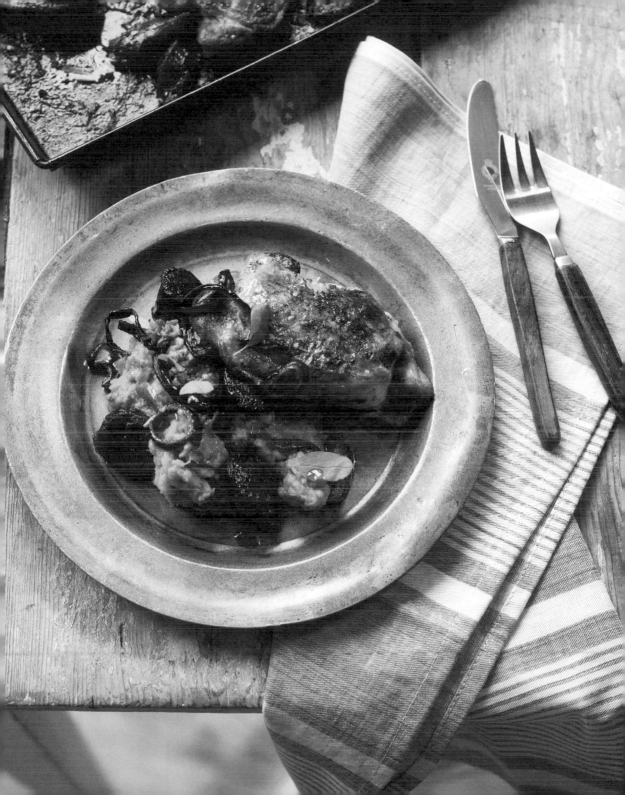

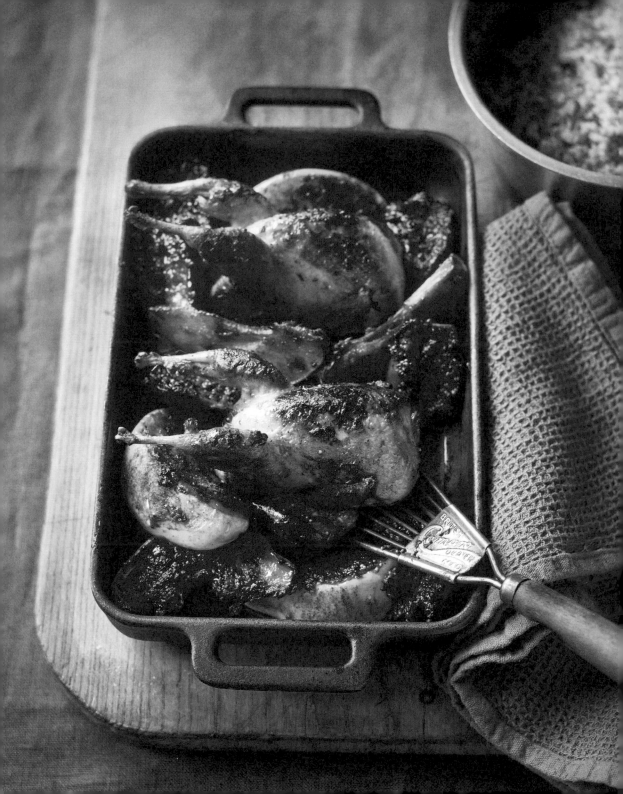

When I was growing up in Ireland in the 80s and 90s, before the 'Celtic Tiger's' economic surge hit, bringing with it cheap world travel and the resulting influence on food, there was a culture of 'meat and two veg'. This consisted of blandly seasoned, over-cooked meat ('boiled elephant' as my grandfather called it), served with two vegetables. Luckily my mother's cooking was more adventurous so I escaped this ordeal, but I had enough run-ins with the 'boiled elephant' and soggy vegetables at friends' houses or country pubs to put me off for life, and to long for the exotic tastes of afar. And this dish is precisely that. The quail is anything but bland with the ginger, garlic and cinnamon, and really moist, languishing with juicy quince and figs in maple syrup.

roast quail with quince & figs

3 garlic cloves, peeled

2.5-cm/1-inch knob of fresh ginger, peeled and chopped

sea salt

2 teaspoons dark soy sauce (if you have coeliac disease, use tamari soy sauce and check the label to make sure it is gluten-free)

extra virgin olive oil

4 quail

2 quince

3 tablespoons pure maple syrup

4 fresh figs, torn into chunks

2 teaspoons ground cinnamon

quinoa and light salad, to serve

Serves 4

Using a pestle and mortar or food processor, pound together the garlic, ginger and a pinch of salt. Mix in the soy sauce and 2 tablespoons oil. Coat the quails in the paste, pushing some underneath the skin but being careful not to tear it. Marinate for a few hours if you have time, but certainly no less than 30 minutes.

Preheat the oven to 200°C (400°F) Gas 6.

Heat 1 tablespoon oil in a large saucepan until very hot, then reduce the heat a little, add all the quail (reserving any excess marinade) and brown the skin all over, turning with tongs as you go. This will only take a few minutes. Transfer to a roasting pan.

Cut the quince into quarters and remove the cores. Heat a little oil in a pan, add the reserved marinade, the quince, cinnamon and 2 tablespoons of the maple syrup. Cook until the quince begin to become tender, then add the figs and cook for 1 minute. You may need to add a little water to aid cooking.

Add the quince and figs to the roasting pan, drizzle over the remaining maple syrup and roast in the preheated oven for 15–20 minutes depending on the size of the quail.

Serve with quinoa and a light salad.

Guilt-free because...

Figs are wonderful if you suffer from constipation, as their high fibre content is a helpful way to get things moving again! They are high in potassium, which helps to balance electrolytes if you have too much salt in your diet.

Figs also have more calcium per 100 g/3½ oz. than whole milk, so they are great bone builders.

The best meatballs I have ever eaten are Spanish 'albondigas', which were cooked for me and my family by a great friend of ours from Spain. Moist, full of flavour from the Moorish spices and deeply satisfying, they are the perfect sharing dish.

spanish meatballs

extra virgin olive oil
sea salt and freshly
    ground black pepper
1 tablespoon freshly
    chopped parsley
bread or quinoa, to serve

Meatballs
2 teaspoons cumin seeds
2 teaspoons coriander
    seeds
1 clove
250 g/9 oz. minced/
    ground beef
200 g/7 oz. minced/
    ground veal
2 teaspoons grated
    nutmeg
2 teaspoons ground
    cinnamon
4 garlic cloves, crushed
6 Medjool dates, pitted
    and finely chopped

1 red chilli, seeded and
    finely chopped
2 eggs, lightly beaten

Tomato Sauce
1 teaspoon cumin seeds
2 red onions, halved and
    sliced
4 garlic cloves, crushed
1 teaspoon ground
    cinnamon
1 teaspoon sweet
    smoked paprika
100 ml/scant ½ cup
    red wine
2 x 400-g/14-oz. cans
    chopped tomatoes
2 dried bay leaves
6 sprigs fresh marjoram
    or oregano
1 tablespoon pure maple
    syrup

Serves 6

To make the meatballs, put the cumin, coriander and clove in a dry pan and toast for 1–2 minutes until you can smell the aromas wafting up from the pan. Pound to a powder using a pestle and mortar.

Put the beef, veal, toasted spices, nutmeg, cinnamon, garlic, dates, chilli and eggs in a food processor, season with a good pinch of salt and pepper and process until smooth. Cover and allow to rest in the fridge for 30 minutes.

Shape the meat mixture into 3–4-cm/1½-inch meatballs with your hands and refrigerate again.

Meanwhile, to make the tomato sauce, toast and grind the cumin seeds as above. In the same pan, heat 2 tablespoons oil over medium heat. Add the onions and cook until translucent. If they are beginning to colour, turn down the heat a little and stir. Add the garlic, a good pinch of salt and pepper, toasted cumin, cinnamon and paprika and cook for a few minutes to release all the flavours, but do not allow the garlic to burn. Add the wine, turn the heat up to high and boil for 1–2 minutes until the wine has almost entirely evaporated. Add the chopped tomatoes and bay leaves, turn the heat down and simmer for 20 minutes, stirring occasionally.

Finally, add the marjoram or oregano and maple syrup. Season to taste. Some canned tomatoes can be quite bitter, in which case you can add another tablespoonful or 2 of maple syrup to achieve a well rounded taste.

Remove the meatballs from the fridge and add to the sauce. Simmer gently for about 20 minutes or until they are cooked through. If the sauce reduces down too much, you can add a little water.

Sprinkle the parsley over, then serve with torn bread to mop up all the juices, or on a bed of quinoa.

Guilt-free because…

Red chilli added to a dish does more than give a satisfying 'kick' to the taste buds. A randomized trial using both men and women found that eating fresh chilli protected blood fats (e.g. cholesterol and triglycerides) from oxidation. Oxidation of fats within the blood is one of the first steps in the development of atherosclerosis (hardening of the arteries), so having spicy dishes is a great way of promoting a healthy cardiovascular system.

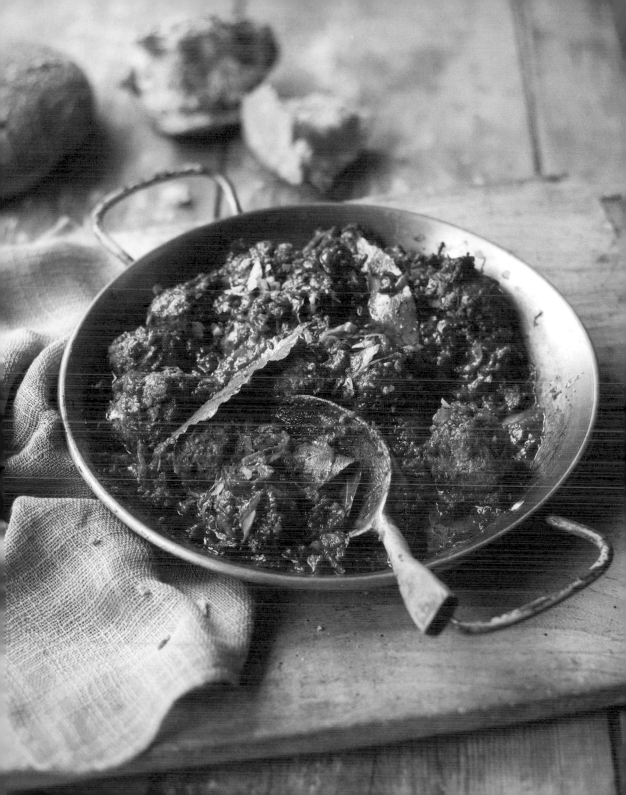

light & fresh

Perfect for a light dinner, summer lunch outside or as a starter or side dish for a dinner party, all of the recipes in this chapter are light and fresh and full of flavour. Check out what's on offer at your local farmers' market, as they are a great source of fresh seasonal produce and you rarely have to do much to it to make it taste good.

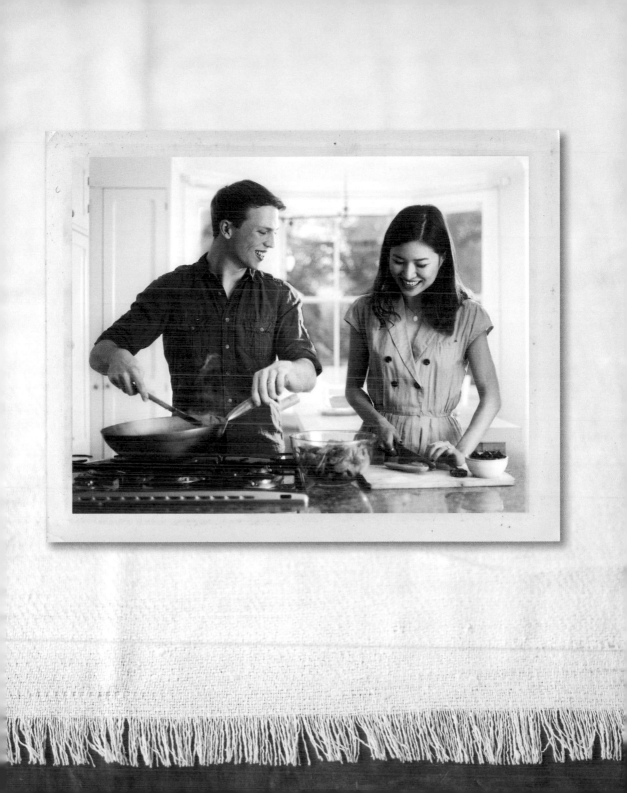

This simple combination of vegetables is a good example of how little you have to do with produce that is really fresh and in season. Personally, I love eating this as a side dish with fish, or with a pile of sweet potato mash.

globe artichoke, fennel & rocket

3 globe artichokes
bunch of fresh thyme
bunch of fresh oregano
sea salt and freshly
    ground black pepper
3 fennel bulbs
2 lemons
extra virgin olive oil
100 g/3½ oz. rocket/
    arugula leaves
1 tablespoon freshly
    chopped parsley

Serves 4

Preheat the oven to 200°C (400°F) Gas 6.

Fill a saucepan with enough water to just cover the artichokes (but don't add the artichokes yet) and bring to the boil. Cut the stalks off the artichokes leaving about 4 cm/1½ inches in length from the base. With a small, serrated knife, cut the top quarter of the artichoke off so that you come down to the top of the choke. Pull off the outer layers of tough leaves until you get to the inner, pale leaves of the heart. Peel the stalk and the base of the artichoke so that there is no outer layer of skin left on at all. Now cut the artichokes in half lengthways through the stalk and remove the prickly inner choke with a teaspoon. Have a lemon ready to squeeze over the skin in order to prevent it from discolouring.

Put the prepared artichokes, thyme, oregano and about 2 teaspoons of salt into the pan of boiling water.

Reduce the heat a little and simmer until the artichokes are very tender and a sharp knife can be easily inserted. In order to keep the artichokes submerged and prevent them from discolouring, place a heatproof plate or lid directly on the surface of the water.

Meanwhile, cut the base and tops off the fennel bulbs and remove the tough outer layer. Cut into quarters, then toss with at least 2 tablespoons of oil in a bowl until well coated. Season with a good pinch of salt and transfer to a baking sheet. Peel the zest off 1 lemon in large pieces, cut the lemon in half, then add all of it to the fennel. Cover with foil and bake in the preheated oven for about 35 minutes (more for large bulbs), until quite soft. A sharp knife should glide into the middle without any resistance. Remove the foil and roast for a further 10 minutes or until they colour a little bit.

Once the artichokes and fennel are ready, grate the zest from the second lemon and add most of it to the vegetables with a drizzle of olive oil. Toss the rocket/arugula with the remaining lemon zest, the juice of ½ lemon some salt and oil. Plate it up with the fennel and artichokes nestled into the leaves. Scatter over the chopped parsley and drizzle with a little more oil.

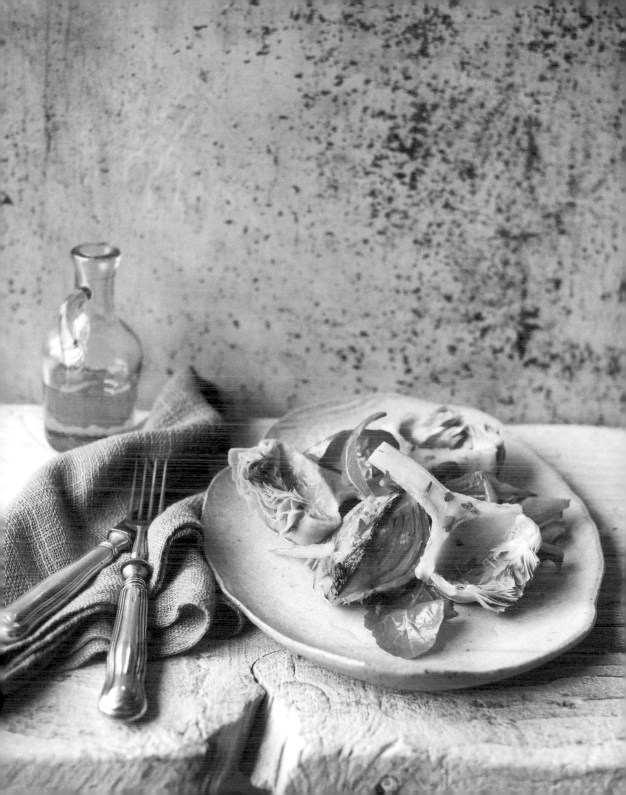

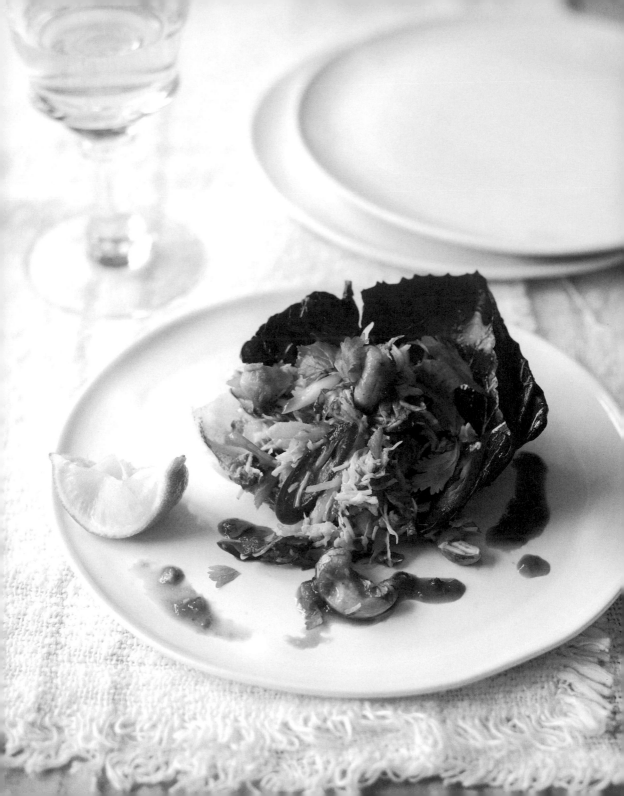

Crab is a wonderful vehicle for other ingredients, which is perfect for this salad, as it is packed full of punchy Thai flavours — coriander/cilantro, fish sauce, lime and chilli. The mango and coconut give it a subtle sweetness that always reminds me of warm summer days, when it makes the ideal dish for a barbecue party or alfresco lunch.

crab with mango & coconut

30 g/¼ cup cashews
2 garlic cloves
thumb-size piece of fresh ginger, peeled and chopped
2 sweet chillies, seeded (if you are using normal red chillies, only use 1½ chillies as they have more heat than the sweet variety)
1 tablespoon nam pla fish sauce
3 teaspoons coconut palm sugar
2 limes (juice of ½ lime and the rest cut into wedges for serving)

300 g/10½ oz. crab meat, picked through for shells
1 firm, slightly under-ripe mango, peeled, pitted and cut into fine strips
handful of fresh coriander/cilantro leaves
2 spring onions/scallions, sliced on the diagonal
a few radicchio leaves or leaves of your choice
extra virgin olive oil
½ lemon
sea salt
2 tablespoons shaved or desiccated dried coconut

Serves 4

Preheat the oven to 180°C (350°F) Gas 4.

Roast the cashews on a baking sheet in the preheated oven for about 10 minutes or until they begin to colour. Watch carefully, as they burn alarmingly quickly!

Using a pestle and mortar, pound the garlic, ginger and chillies (keeping ½ chilli aside for serving) until you get a paste. Add the fish sauce, coconut sugar and lime juice. Combine until well blended.

Squeeze any excess liquid out of the picked crab. In a large bowl, combine the crab, mango, coriander/cilantro (leaving some aside for serving), spring onions/scallions and roasted cashews. Add the sauce and mix gently.

Dress the radicchio leaves with a little oil, a squeeze of lemon juice and a pinch of salt. Pile the crab mixture on top of the leaves and finish off with the coconut and reserved coriander/cilantro and chilli, sliced. Serve with lime wedges.

Guilt-free because...

Mango is a revered fruit in Asia, not only for its sweet, tangy taste but also for its health benefits. It contains enzymes similar to papain in papayas, which are helpful for digestive discomfort.

Lab testing of mangoes has shown the juice to be effective at killing viruses and cancer cells. This is thought to be due to its high levels of phenols, which have antioxidant and anti-cancer properties. Phenols include quercetin, isoquercitrin and the particular type most evident in mango flesh: gallic acid.

Up until my teens, I wouldn't touch fish. I have a vague memory of being force-fed fish fingers when I said I didn't like them (who could blame me?) and that very nearly put me off for life. Years later, my sister insisted I try her halibut dish, saying it was meaty and not in the least bit fishy. That was the beginning of my fish rehabilitation and halibut remains one of my favourites. However, it is now listed as endangered, so it is crucial to buy only sustainably caught halibut. Look for the blue MSC label or ask your fishmonger.

halibut with fennel, olives & tomato

3 fennel bulbs
extra virgin olive oil
sea salt and freshly
   ground black pepper
1 lemon
250 g/8 oz. plum
   tomatoes
red wine vinegar
bunch of fresh parsley,
   finely chopped
2 garlic cloves, finely
   chopped
4 x 150-g/5-oz. halibut
   fillets, skin on
2 tablespoons black and
   green olives, pitted
   (I like the French
   Picholine and Niçoise
   varieties)

Serves 4

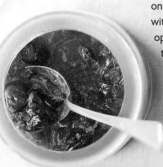

Preheat the oven to 200°C (400°F) Gas 6.

Cut the base and tops off the fennel bulbs and remove the tough outer layer. Cut into quarters, then toss with at least 2 tablespoons oil in a bowl until well coated. Season with a good pinch of salt and transfer to a baking sheet. Peel the zest off 1 lemon in large pieces and add to the fennel. Cover with foil and bake in the preheated oven for about 35 minutes (more for large bulbs), until quite soft. A sharp knife should glide into the middle without any resistance. Remove the foil and roast for a further 10 minutes or until they colour a little bit.

Toss the tomatoes in enough oil to coat them liberally, season well with salt and 1 tablespoon vinegar. Roast them on a separate baking sheet in the oven with the fennel until the skins pop open – about 15 minutes. Time it so that the fennel and tomatoes both finish cooking around the same time.

While the vegetables are roasting, combine the parsley and garlic with enough oil – about 5 tablespoons – to make a thick parsley oil. Add the olives and season with a pinch of salt.

When the vegetables have finished roasting, turn the oven off and let them sit in the residual heat.

Put 2 saucepans over medium heat and add 1 tablespoon oil to each. Season the halibut fillets with salt and pepper and drizzle oil over both sides of the fillet. Once the pans are hot, place 2 halibut fillets in each pan, skin side down. Let them sizzle for about 2–3 minutes, then turn over and cook for another 2–3 minutes (depending on the thickness of your fillet) until they are just cooked through.

Serve the fennel with the tomatoes dotted around it. Place a halibut fillet on top, skin side up. Stir the parsley oil and spoon a good amount over the fish, fennel and tomatoes, making sure to get the olives in too. Serve immediately.

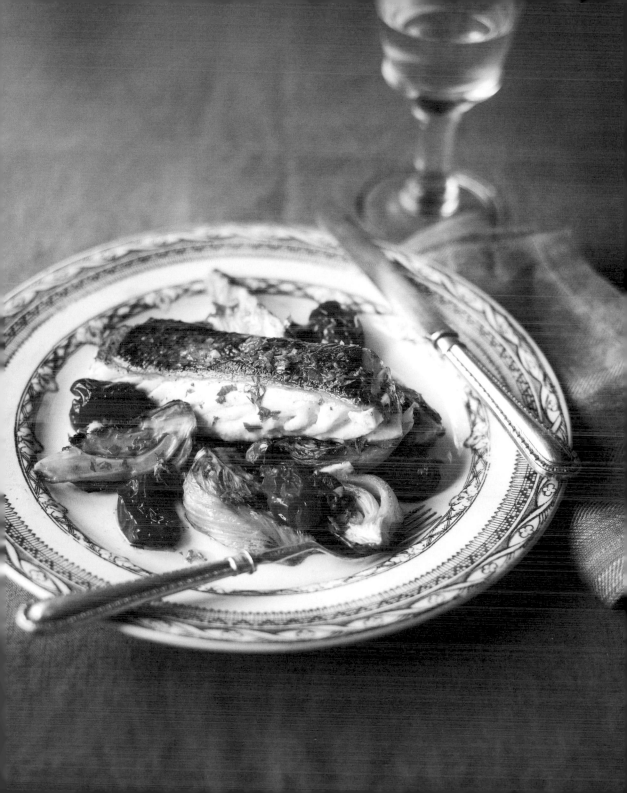

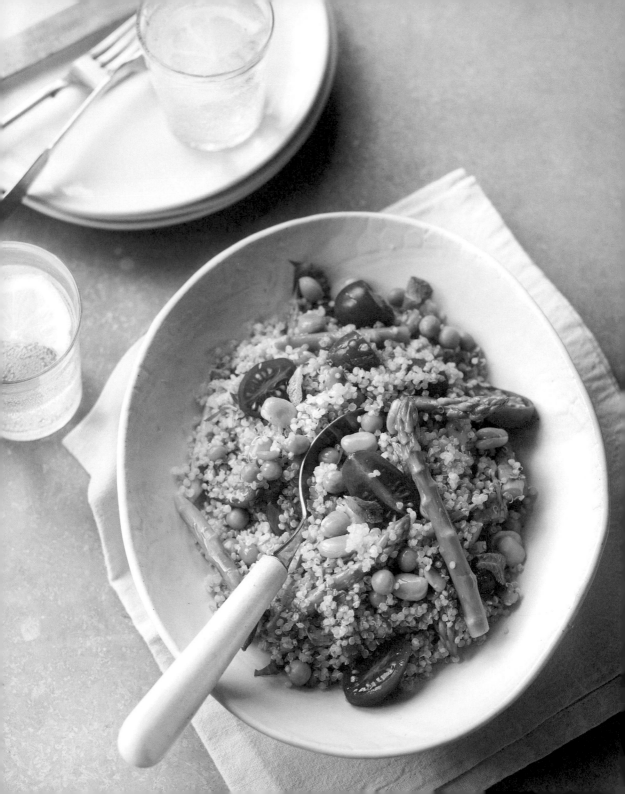

It is only in the last few years that quinoa has found its place on the shelves of most supermarkets, and despite a growth in its popularity, I still think its taste and nutritional benefits remain largely unknown. Quinoa should really be just as popular as rice or pasta for your daily cooking needs, if not more so. This dish is a celebration of new-season spring vegetables, using the ones that I enjoy most at this time of year. At other times of year you can find asparagus ranging from white to crimson — they are great for adding a splash of colour.

quinoa with new-season beans, peas & asparagus

300 g/1½ cups quinoa
2 teaspoons bouillon
    stock powder
sea salt and freshly
    ground black pepper
12 asparagus spears,
    chopped in half
200 g/2 cups shelled
    broad/fava beans
200 g/2 cups peas
large handful of fresh mint
handful of fresh parsley
handful of cherry
    tomatoes, halved
grated zest and juice of
    1 lemon
200 ml/¾ cup extra virgin
    olive oil
1 tablespoon maple syrup
1 tablespoon
    pomegranate molasses
    (or balsamic vinegar)

Serves 6

Put the quinoa and bouillon powder in a saucepan and cover with just under double its volume of water. Bring to the boil, then reduce the heat to low and place the lid on top. Cook for about 12 minutes until all the water has been absorbed. Turn off the heat, remove the lid and let any remaining water evaporate. Remove to a wide plate or tray and allow to cool.

Meanwhile, bring a pan of water to the boil (just enough to cover each set of vegetables you are cooking) and add 2 teaspoons salt. Cook the asparagus, beans and peas separately until just tender – about 3–4 minutes for each. You still want them to have a bit of bite.

Once the beans are cooked, they need to have their outer cases removed. This is a bit of a nightmare but the end result is truly worth it, for the colour if for nothing else. I like to delegate jobs to family or friends who might be joining me for dinner, and this is the perfect job for them! Simply slide the pale case off each bean and discard.

Roughly chop the herbs.

In a large bowl, gently but thoroughly mix the quinoa, asparagus, beans, peas, tomatoes and herbs, reserving some of the herbs for serving. Add the lemon zest and juice, oil, maple syrup, molasses, salt and pepper. Mix again, taste and adjust the seasoning if necessary.

Serve in a large dish with the remaining herbs sprinkled on top. Finish off with a drizzle of oil. Simple, but magnificent.

Guilt-free because…

Quinoa is a fantastic source of easily digested protein – 200 g/ 1 cup quinoa provides 3 g more protein than an egg, plus it supplies all 8 of the essential amino acids, so it is a 'complete' protein for vegetarians and meat-eaters alike.

I was asked to cook for a dinner party last year and when I suggested lentils as a pairing for the meat, the host laughed at me! Her feeling was that lentils were 'a bit too hippy, vegan' for her, and that her guests would rather have potato. The problem is, people don't realize that with lentils it is all about the seasoning – lashings of olive oil, lemon juice and salt. Here sun-dried tomatoes, lentils and aubergine/eggplant make a delicious yet simple accompaniment to fish or meat.

aubergine, puy lentils & sun-dried tomatoes with mint oil

300 g/1½ cups Puy lentils (or other green lentils)
extra virgin olive oil
1 red onion, finely chopped
2 garlic cloves, crushed
450 ml/2 cups vegetable stock (or water, a carrot, ½ onion, celery stalk, bay leaf and thyme in the lentils to make your own stock as they cook)
3 aubergines/eggplants, topped, tailed and cut into ¼-cm/½-inch slices
sea salt and freshly ground black pepper
grated zest of 1 lemon and juice of ½
100 g/⅔ cup sun-dried tomatoes
1 tablespoon agave syrup
1 tablespoon red wine vinegar
1 tablespoon dark soy sauce (if you have coeliac disease, use tamari soy sauce and check the label to make sure it is gluten-free)
big handful of fresh mint leaves

Serves 4

Wash and drain the lentils.

Heat 2 tablespoons oil in a large, heavy-bottomed, lidded casserole dish over medium heat. Turn down the heat a little, add the onion and fry until soft and translucent but not coloured. Add the garlic and fry for 1 minute. Add the lentils and stir well. Pour the vegetable stock in and bring to the boil. Reduce the heat, simmer, then cover with the lid and cook for 25 minutes or until the lentils are tender and have absorbed most of the stock.

Meanwhile, heat a large, dry stovetop grill pan over medium heat until hot. Using a pastry brush, coat the aubergine/eggplant slices with oil on both sides. Place them on the pan and fry for a few minutes. Check they have gone a golden brown and then flip over and fry for another few minutes until golden. They should be soft to the touch. Remove to a plate and season with salt. Drizzle over the agave syrup and plenty of oil. (The quality of the oil is key here, as the aubergine really soaks it all up so you will really be able to taste it.)

When the lentils are done, drain them of all but a few tablespoons of the cooking liquid. While they are still hot, season with the lemon zest and juice, vinegar and soy sauce and a few glugs of oil. Mix well and allow to cool slightly. Taste it when it is at room temperature and season if necessary. Add the tomatoes and mix together.

Finely chop the mint leaves (reserving a few for serving) and combine with enough oil to make a dense mint oil. To serve, nestle the aubergine/eggplant slices among the lentils, drizzle over the mint oil and scatter with the remaining leaves.

Guilt-free because…

Puy lentils have a wonderful 'meaty' texture yet contain no cholesterol, are high in protein and have a very low glycaemic index, which means they release energy at a slow and steady rate. They are a good source of fibre, magnesium, potassium and zinc.

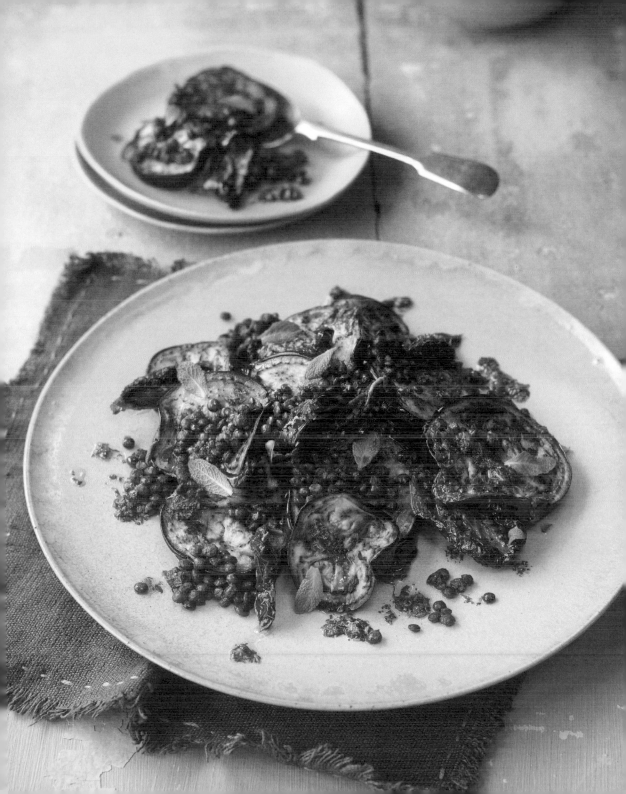

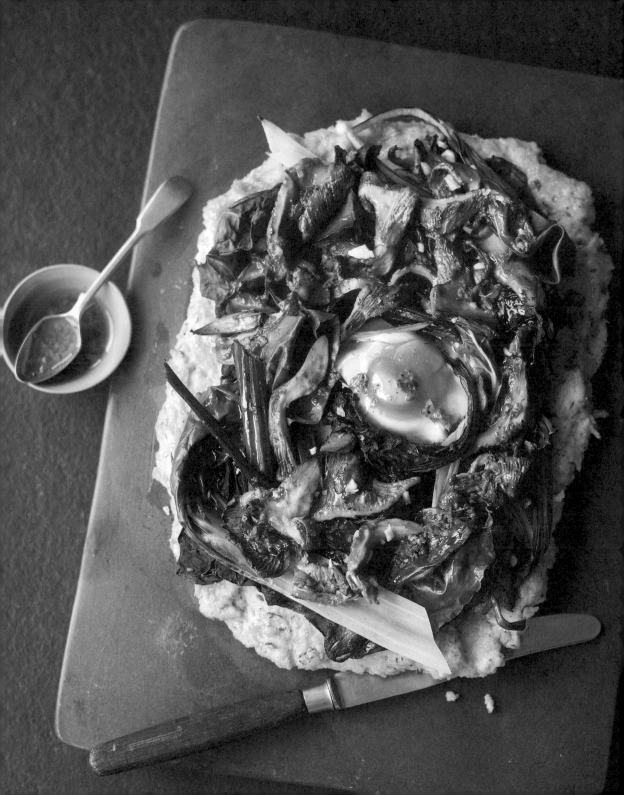

Polenta can be served in soft and gloopy form, or it can be cooked a little further to dry it out and then grilled/broiled to achieve a firmer, breadier base layer. Either way it can be dreadfully bland if it's not seasoned generously. I love this grilled/broiled version, as it soaks up all the juices from the toppings served with it and it has a satisfying texture. Totally guilt free, as it is made from corn, this is a fantastic lunch or dinner dish to share with friends.

polenta pizza

2 teaspoons bouillon
  stock powder
200 g/1⅓ cups polenta/
  yellow cornmeal
grated zest and juice of
  1 lemon
6 garlic cloves, crushed
sea salt and freshly
  ground black pepper
1 tablespoon fresh thyme
  leaves
1 head of rainbow or
  Swiss chard
extra virgin olive oil
200 g/7 oz. girolle/
  golden chanterelle
  mushrooms
1 tablespoon freshly
  chopped parsley
1 egg
bunch of fresh marjoram

large baking sheet, oiled

Serves 6

Bring 1 litre/4 cups water to the boil and add the bouillon powder. Reduce the heat and slowly pour in the polenta/cornmeal, whisking all the time until blended. Reduce the heat to its lowest setting, add half the lemon zest and juice, 4 of the crushed garlic cloves, the thyme and a good pinch of salt and pepper and gently cook, stirring occasionally, for about 45 minutes or until the polenta pulls away from the side of the pan and is very thick.

Meanwhile, bring another pan of water to the boil. Add 1 teaspoon salt and boil the chard for about 3–4 minutes until the thick part is just tender, but not limp. If the root end of the chard is very thick, separate it from the leaves and boil each part separately until just tender. Remove, drain and season with some salt and oil.

In the meantime, don't forget to stir the polenta!

Heat 2 tablespoons oil in another pan over medium–high heat. Fry the mushrooms for about 2 minutes or until just golden and tender. Add 1 of the crushed garlic cloves and stir for 30 seconds to release the garlic flavour, but don't let it burn. Transfer to a bowl, toss with the parsley and season with

salt, the remaining lemon zest and juice, and some olive oil.

When the polenta is ready, transfer to the prepared baking sheet and spread out to a thickness of about 2 cm/¾ inch. Allow to cool and firm up for 30 minutes.

Preheat the grill/broiler.

Scatter the mushrooms and chard over the top of the polenta. Crack an egg carefully into the middle and grill/broil for about 4–5 minutes or until the egg is cooked.

Meanwhile, pull the leaves off the marjoram stalks and finely chop. Mix the chopped leaves with the last crushed garlic clove and mix with enough oil to form a loose marjoram oil.

Remove the polenta from the grill/broiler, slide onto a board and drizzle the marjoram oil over the top. Serve immediately.

This is such a simple yet effective dish and is great for diving into and getting your hands dirty with a big group of friends. The Nam Jim is a wonderfully vibrant Thai sauce that makes these totally addictive. Make sure you use the roots of the coriander/cilantro and not the leaves, as this is where all the flavour is. I have used coconut palm sugar here, as it is far better for you than other sugars. It has been used for hundreds of years in Southeast Asian cooking. Don't confuse it with Thai palm sugar, which comes in white hard blobs.

charred shrimp with nam jim

roots of 1 bunch of
   coriander/cilantro
2 garlic cloves
2.5 cm/1 inch fresh
   ginger
1 large red chilli, seeded,
   plus extra slices,
   to serve
1 tablespoon coconut
   palm sugar
sea salt
2 teaspoons fish sauce
juice of 1 lime
8 king prawns/jumbo
   shrimp, shell on

Serves 3–4

Using a pestle and mortar, pound the coriander/cilantro roots, garlic, ginger and chilli until you get a paste. This will take a few minutes of fairly aggressive pounding! The skin of the chilli will also come loose so when that happens, you should pick it out and discard it.

Add the sugar and pound, then add a little salt, the fish sauce and lime juice. Mix together and taste. This Nam Jim is so full of flavour that it should almost sing out at you, with each ingredient holding its own. Adjust it ever so slightly until you get the right balance.

Heat a stovetop grill pan over high heat. Cut the prawns/shrimp lengthways down the middle of the belly, so you have nice long halves. Place them, flesh side down, on the dry pan, cook for 2 minutes, then flip them over and cook for another 2 minutes.

Once cooked, tangle the prawns/shrimp together on a plate with some coriander/cilantro leaves and extra chilli slices scattered over. Drizzle with Nam Jim and serve.

Guilt-free because…

Coconut palm sugar may soon become the sweetener of choice for those who care about their health. As it is derived from the sap of the cut flower buds of the coconut tree, it is classified as a whole food and is not synthesized in a lab like artificial sweeteners are. It has a very low GI of 35–54 whereas normal table sugar has a GI of 65–100 per serving. It is particularly high in the amino acid glutamine, which is involved in more metabolic processes than any other amino acid. It also contains inositol, a B-complex nutrient that creates a calming effect on the body and has proved useful in cases of depression and panic attacks.

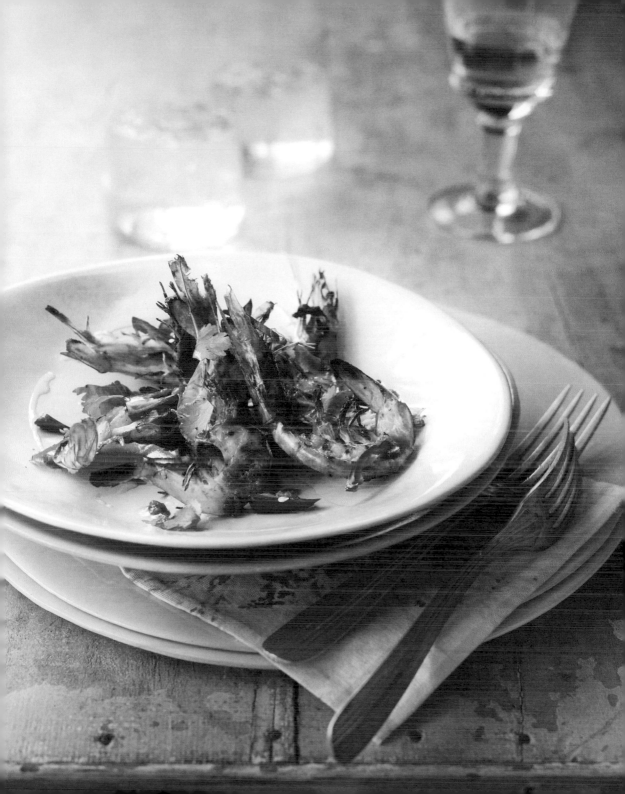

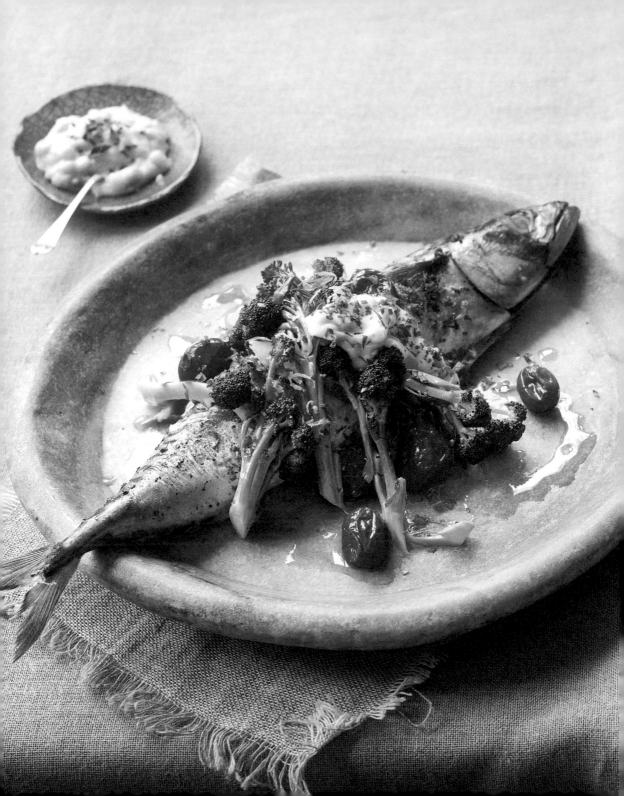

I love mackerel. It is easy to cook, tastes great, is dirt-cheap and is often the perfect size for one person. It does have to be totally fresh though, so try to buy it from a place you can trust. Look out for cloudy eyes – if it is really fresh, they will be crystal clear and glassy in appearance. With depleting fish stocks a very serious issue, I urge you all to try to buy only certified sustainable fish. Check the label or tag, or if you shop at a fishmonger's, ask the person at the counter.

mackerel with sprouting broccoli, cherry tomatoes & almond aïoli

6 tablespoons good extra
   virgin olive oil
20 cherry tomatoes –
   as ripe and red as you
   can find
sea salt and freshly
   ground black pepper
1 tablespoon red wine
   vinegar
grated zest and juice
   of ½ lemon
4 small mackerel (or
   2 large), gutted and
   cleaned
300 g/10 oz. sprouting
   broccoli
small bunch of fresh
   parsley, finely chopped

Almond Aïoli
Wholegrain Mustard
   Mayonnaise recipe
   (page 90) but follow
   method here
3 garlic cloves, crushed
50 g/⅓ cup blanched
   almonds

Serves 4

To make the almond aïoli, make a mayonnaise base following the recipe on page 90, but add the crushed garlic at the beginning before you start whisking in the oil, and omit the wholegrain mustard.

Preheat the oven to 180°C (350°F) Gas 4.

Roast the almonds in the preheated oven for about 8 minutes or until they turn a shade darker. Leave the oven on. Using a pestle and mortar, bash the almonds roughly so they are still chunky – you do not want to grind them to a powder – as the coarse texture is wonderful with the fish. Stir them through the aïoli.

Toss the tomatoes in enough oil to coat them and season generously with

salt and the vinegar. Roast on a baking sheet for about 15 minutes or until the skins burst open. Keep warm.

Meanwhile, steam the broccoli for 3–4 minutes or until it has turned a vibrant shade of emerald green. Season with a little salt, the lemon zest and juice and a good drizzle of oil.

Score the fish 3 times on each side, brush with oil and season with salt and pepper. Heat a frying pan over medium heat and fry the fish for 3–4 minutes on one side (depending on their size and thickness) without moving them. Flip over and fry for 3–4 minutes again.

Put each mackerel on a plate, tangle the broccoli and tomatoes on top and dollop a big spoonful of the almond aïoli over. Sprinkle with the parsley.

Guilt-free because…

Mackerel is an oily fish, so it is high in health-promoting essential fatty acids. It is great for cardiovascular health as it helps to reduce LDL (bad) cholesterol while also providing 'brain food' to improve concentration and memory. King Mackerel has higher levels of mercury contamination so should be avoided during pregnancy.

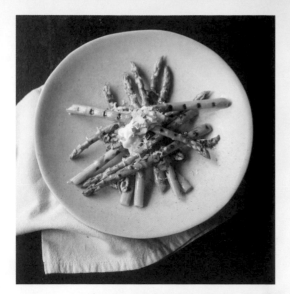

When I manage to get my hands on beautifully fresh, in-season vegetables I prefer not to mess around with them too much, which is how I came up with with this asparagus dish. The cannellini bean recipe came together by accident while on holiday in France. We had lots of cannellini beans, avocados and mint to use up, so we made a giant salad. Together with meatballs or falafel, this is ideal for a casual lunch or dinner.

chargrilled asparagus
with walnut mayonnaise

Wholegrain Mustard
 Mayonnaise recipe
 (page 90), omitting the
 wholegrain mustard
 and using walnut oil
 instead of sunflower
bunch of asparagus spears
extra virgin olive oil

grated zest of ½ lemon
sea salt
small handful of walnuts,
 fresh from the shell
a little freshly chopped
 parsley

Serves 2–4

Heat a stovetop grill pan over high heat. Snap the bases off the asparagus spears where they naturally break. Toss the asparagus in a few drops of oil so that they are lightly coated.

Grill the asparagus for about 3 minutes depending on the thickness. Turn them now and again to get an even char. You want the asparagus to still retain a bit of bite.

Pile the asparagus up on a plate and scatter over some lemon zest and salt. Put a big blob of the walnut mayonnaise on top, scatter over the walnuts and parsley and drizzle over some olive oil.

cannellini bean,
avocado & mint

2 x 400-g/14-oz. cans
 cannellini beans (buying
 dried beans, soaking
 them and cooking them
 is definitely better and
 cheaper, but when you
 don't have time, canned
 beans are fine)
2 large avocados
4 spring onions/scallions
 sliced on the diagonal

good handful of fresh
 mint leaves, torn if they
 are very big
1 garlic clove, crushed
grated zest and fresh juice
 of 1 lemon
4 tablespoons extra virgin
 olive oil
sea salt and freshly
 ground black pepper

Serves 4–6

Drain and rinse the beans and place in a bowl. Cut the avocados in half, remove the stones and spoon the flesh out of the skin. Slice lengthways and add to the bowl. Add the spring onions/scallions, mint leaves, garlic, lemon zest and juice, and oil. Mix together and season to taste with salt and pepper. If it does not taste exciting, add more lemon zest, salt and oil.

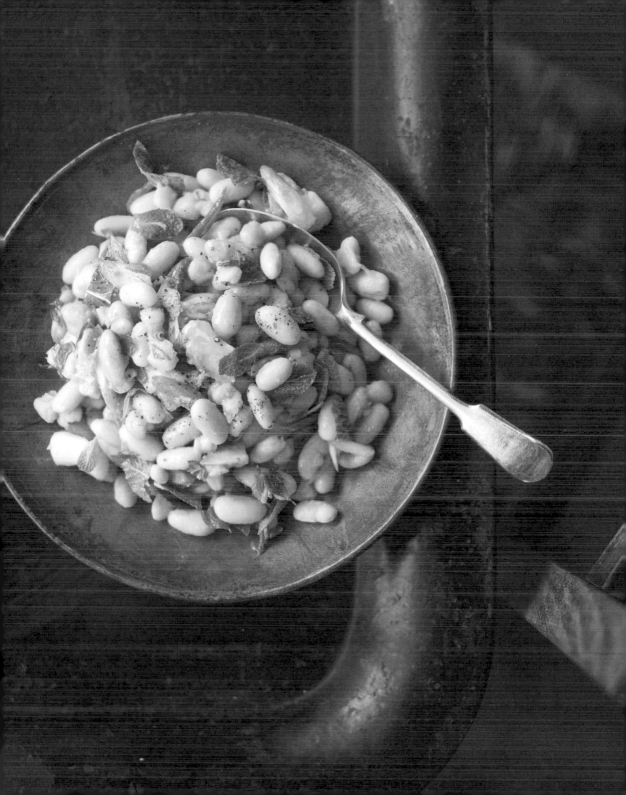

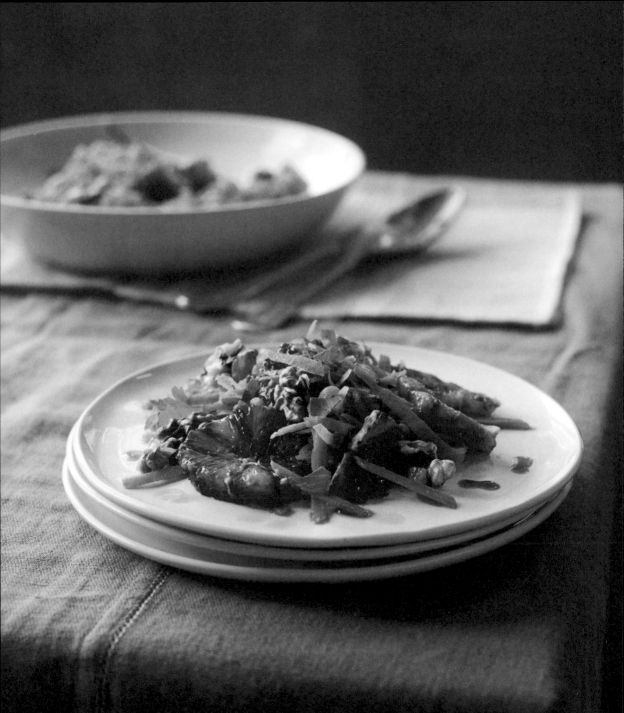

The colour of this blood orange salad is enough to win anyone over, but it is full of flavour as well. It's perfect as a side or with a number of other salads, all sumptuously laid out together. Get your hands on blood oranges while they are in season. The super simple tomato salad celebrates the incredible variety of tomatoes at our fingertips today, which are just as delicious as any you might find on a sun-drenched vine in Italy.

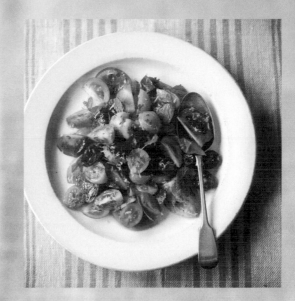

grated carrots, blood orange & walnuts

2 blood oranges
8 large carrots, grated
grated zest and juice of 1 lemon
1 tablespoon maple syrup
1 tablespoon freshly chopped parsley

4 tablespoons extra virgin olive oil
sea salt
2 handfuls of walnuts, fresh from the shell

Serves 6

Cut the top and bottom off the oranges, just down to the flesh, then place the orange on its end, cut side down, and carefully, following the shape of the orange, cut the peel off in strips from top to bottom, making sure you cut off the white pith too. Then turn them on their side and cut them into 1-cm/⅜-inch thick rounds. Do this on a board or somewhere that will catch any orange juice that you inadvertently squeeze out of them; this can be added to the dish too.

Squeeze any excess juice out of the grated carrots to prevent the salad from being too soggy (you can drink any juice you extract). In a large bowl, combine the carrots with all the other ingredients. This should be a punchy, citrussy salad with just enough sweetness from the maple syrup. Let all the flavours combine together for 15 minutes, then taste again, adjust the seasoning if necessary.

heritage tomato salad

any variety of heirloom tomato, eg. San Marzano, Oxheart, Cuban Yellow Grape, Datterini, Camone, Tiger etc. (best bought from farmers' markets: check online for your nearest one)
sea salt

grated zest and juice of 1 lemon
good extra virgin olive oil
red wine vinegar
fresh mint and basil leaves
spelt bread, to mop up the oil and tomato juices!

Serves as many people as you like!

The tomatoes should be room temperature in order for all the flavour to come through, so if you have them in the fridge, take them out well in advance. Give them a quick rinse, then cut them in a variety of ways, from rounds and wedges, to quarters and halves. Lay them all out on a board and season generously with salt, lemon zest and juice, oil and a few drops of vinegar. Season each piece properly but go easy on the vinegar.

Pile them on a plate with the basil and mint intertwined. Season with a little extra salt and oil as you go. Finish with a few leaves on top. Serve with a hunk of spelt bread brushed with a sliced garlic clove.

foods from afar

There is nothing quite like the exotic flavours of afar. From Thai curry and fiery Korean noodles to Japanese tempura and Moroccan tagines, they instantly transport you to another world of mystery and spices. Ethnic ingredients are very easy to get your hands on, so dive into these recipes and bring a taste of the Orient that bit closer to home.

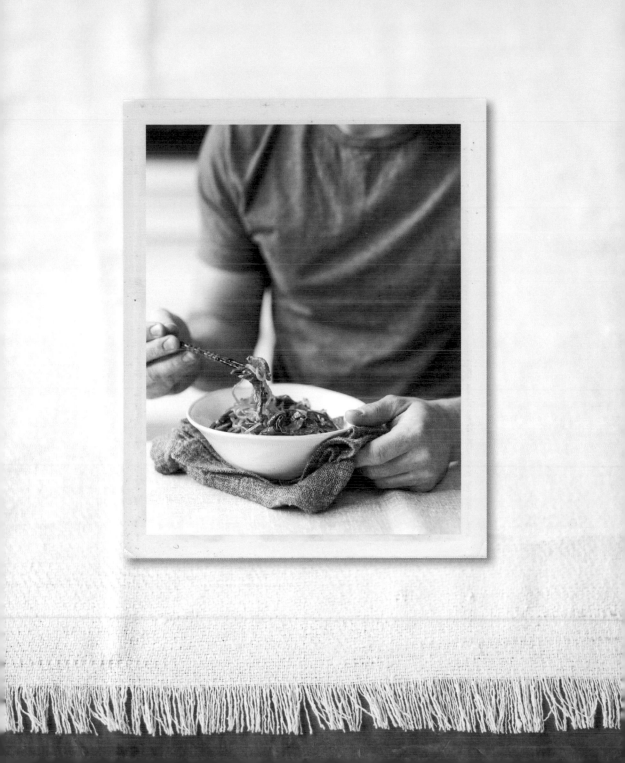

The flavours here vary from deep and complex to clean and fresh all at the same time and would fool anyone into thinking you had spent hours slaving over it. It is a great soup when you are slightly under the weather — the coconut milk soothes while the chilli and galangal blast away any potential viruses. Making your own chicken stock in advance makes a big difference and it can be frozen until you need it.

thai coconut & lemongrass soup
with shrimp

Chicken Stock (optional)
1 chicken carcass
1 celery stick
1 carrot
1 sprig fresh thyme
1 onion, halved
a few fresh parsley stalks
a few black peppercorns

Soup
1 litre/4 cups chicken stock
5 kaffir lime leaves
fresh juice of 2 limes
2 lemongrass sticks, bruised
5-cm/2-inch piece of galangal, thinly sliced (or a smaller amount of fresh ginger)
3 tablespoons nam pla fish sauce
250 ml/1 cup coconut milk
15 prawns/shrimp
3 red chillies, seeded and chopped
handful of fresh coriander/cilantro leaves

Serves 6

To make the chicken stock, put all the ingredients and 2.5 litres/10 cups cold water in a large saucepan and bring to the boil. Reduce the heat and simmer for at least 3 hours. Skim off any fat from the surface and strain off the liquid. If you are stuck for time, you can buy good-quality free-range, organic chicken stock in good supermarkets.

To make the soup, put the chicken stock, lime leaves, lime juice, lemongrass, galangal and fish sauce in a large pan and bring to the boil. Add the coconut milk, prawns/shrimp and chillies (reserving a little for serving) and continue to cook for a couple of minutes until the prawns/shrimp are cooked through. Add the majority of the coriander/cilantro leaves, then check the seasoning and add more fish sauce if necessary. Serve in bowls with the reserved chillies and remaining coriander/cilantro scattered on top.

Guilt-free because...

Lemongrass possesses notable anti-fungal and antibacterial properties, making it a useful ingredient if trying to fight a cold. Its antiseptic qualities have been found to be more effective than some of the strongest antibiotic medications available.

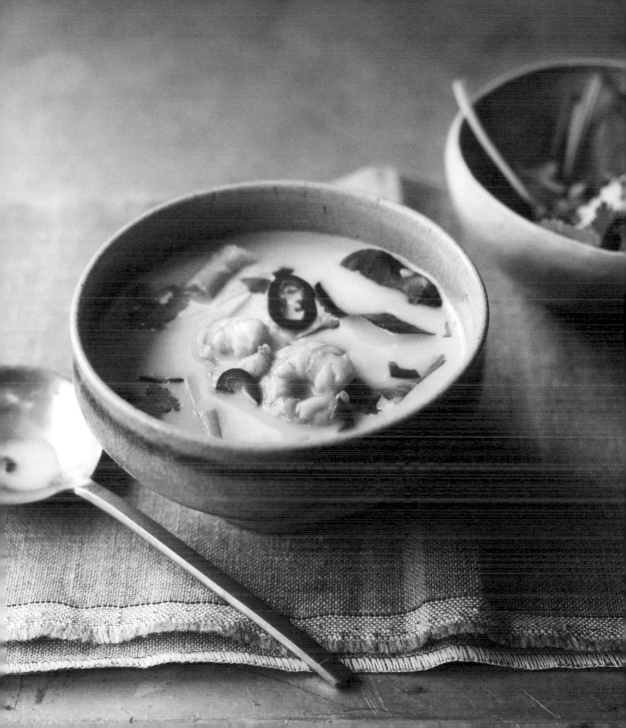

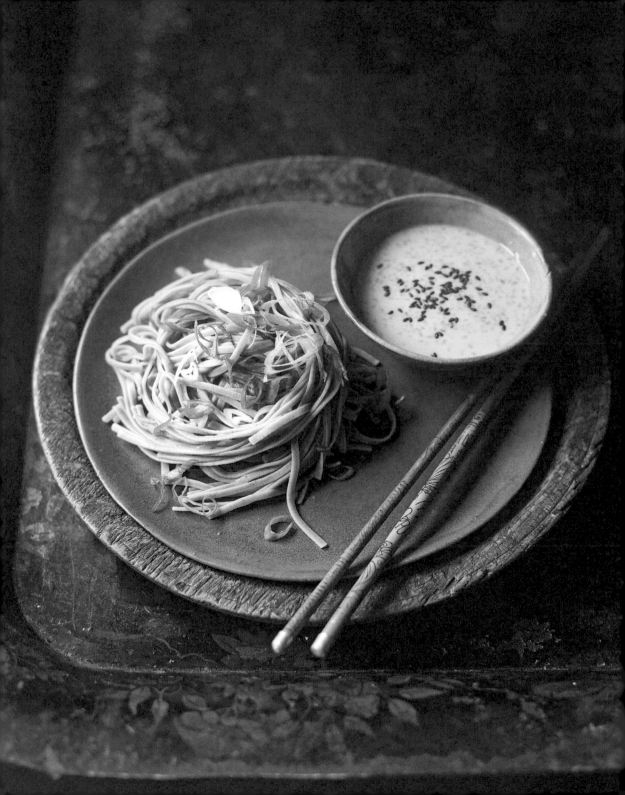

In Japan, these noodle dishes are extremely popular and they are my favourite thing to eat when I'm there. They are very easy to make and a perfect example of Japanese cooking: simple yet elegant. 'Soba' means buckwheat in English, but despite the name, buckwheat contains no wheat or gluten and is really good for you. If you are coeliac, check the ingredients as some brands use a little wheat flour, so you will need to seek out the ones made with 100% buckwheat.

soba noodles with gomadare sesame seed sauce

200 g/6½ oz. buckwheat soba noodles

Gomadare Sauce
2 tablespoons mirin (sweetened rice wine)
1 tablespoon sesame seeds, lightly toasted
2 tablespoons white miso paste
½ tablespoon dark soy sauce (if you have coeliac disease, use tamari soy sauce and check the label to make sure it is gluten-free)
½ tablespoon agave syrup
½ tablespoon rice vinegar
90 ml/6 tablespoons neri goma (Japanese sesame paste) (or tahini mixed with 1 tablespoon toasted sesame oil)
110 ml/½ cup dashi (Japanese stock made from bonito flakes and kombu seaweed)
1 spring onion/scallion, chopped
½ teaspoon black sesame seeds

Serves 2

Bring a saucepan of water to the boil and cook the soba noodles according to the packet instructions.

While they are on, bring the mirin to a fast boil in another saucepan for a minute or so to cook off the alcohol, then remove from the heat.

To make the gomadare sauce, put the sesame seeds, mirin, miso paste, soy sauce, agave syrup, rice vinegar and neri goma in a bowl and mix well. Slowly mix in the dashi, bit by bit, until you reach your desired consistency. Some people like it thicker than others. I find about 110 ml/½ cup dashi gets the perfect consistency.

When the noodles are cooked, drain well and twist into a high mound on each plate with the chopped spring onion/scallion piled on top. Spoon the gomadare sauce into a little bowl beside the noodles and sprinkle the black sesame seeds on top. Serve immediately. To eat, pick up a few noodles with chopsticks and dunk them into the gomadare sauce. I then use a spoon (with the chopsticks) to help me get the noodles from the bowl to my mouth without spraying gomadare onto my unsuspecting dining companions.

Guilt-free because...

Buckwheat is a naturally gluten-free 'grain', derived from a fruit seed. It has received a lot of attention recently for its apparent ability to lower blood sugar levels, which would be great news for diabetics.

A compound in buckwheat called 'd-chiro-inositol' may directly impact glucose metabolism and signalling between cells. It appears the d-chiro-inositol makes the body cells more sensitive to insulin, or in some cases, may even mimic insulin, so the blood sugar levels may be controlled more easily. So far, the research has only been conducted in studies with type 1 diabetes, but scientists are hopeful that the same impressive results will be seen with type 2 diabetes symptoms also.

The heat of wasabi is a wonderful way to liven up mashed potatoes, and the flavour goes so well with soy- and sesame-marinated salmon. As ever, buying sustainably caught fish is crucial if we are to have any left in the sea for future generations. The Marine Stewardship Council website (www.msc.org) has a 'where to buy' section that shows you, worldwide, down to the specific store, where to buy MSC-certified fish.

soy salmon, wasabi mash & bok choi

3 tablespoons dark soy sauce (if you have coeliac disease, use tamari soy sauce and check the label to make sure it is gluten-free)
toasted sesame oil
1 teaspoon agave syrup
fresh juice of 1 lime
2 salmon fillets
500 g/1 lb. potatoes
sea salt
100 g/3½ oz. bok choi, halved lengthways if fat
extra virgin olive oil
100 ml/6 tablespoons soy cream/creamer
1 spring onion/scallion
wasabi paste or powder
1 teaspoon sesame seeds, toasted

Serves 2

Mix together the soy sauce, 1 tablespoon sesame oil, the agave syrup and lime juice in a resealable bag. Place the salmon fillets inside, seal the bag and marinate for at least 20 minutes, or for a few hours if you have the time.

Put the potatoes in a saucepan of cold, salted water. Bring to the boil and cook until just tender but not falling apart. While the potatoes are cooking, bring another pan of water to the boil, add a good pinch of salt and cook the bok choi for a few minutes until just tender. I like them to still have a bit of bite. Drain and season with a drizzle of olive oil and a few drops of sesame oil. Keep warm.

When the potatoes are cooked, drain and place a dry tea towel on top to absorb any remaining moisture. After a few minutes, peel the potatoes by just pulling off the skin. Add the soy cream/creamer, plenty of olive oil and the spring onion/scallion and mash until smooth. You may need more oil as it really does soak in. Season to taste with salt, then cautiously add some wasabi paste or powder. It should be strong enough to definitely taste it though.

When the potatoes are mashed, heat a dry pan over medium heat and add the salmon fillets (reserving the marinade). Fry for 3–4 minutes, then flip over and fry until just cooked through. A minute or so before it is done, add the remaining marinade. Let it bubble, then remove from the heat.

Immediately plate up the wasabi mash, place the salmon on top and nestle the bok choi on top. Sprinkle over some sesame seeds and enjoy.

Guilt-free because...

Salmon is commonly referred to as a 'brain food' due to the high levels of omega-3 fats it contains – namely, EPA and DHA. These forms of omega-3 fats are the type used in the brain and in the nervous system and are extremely important for mood, memory, and cardiovascular, joint and eye health.

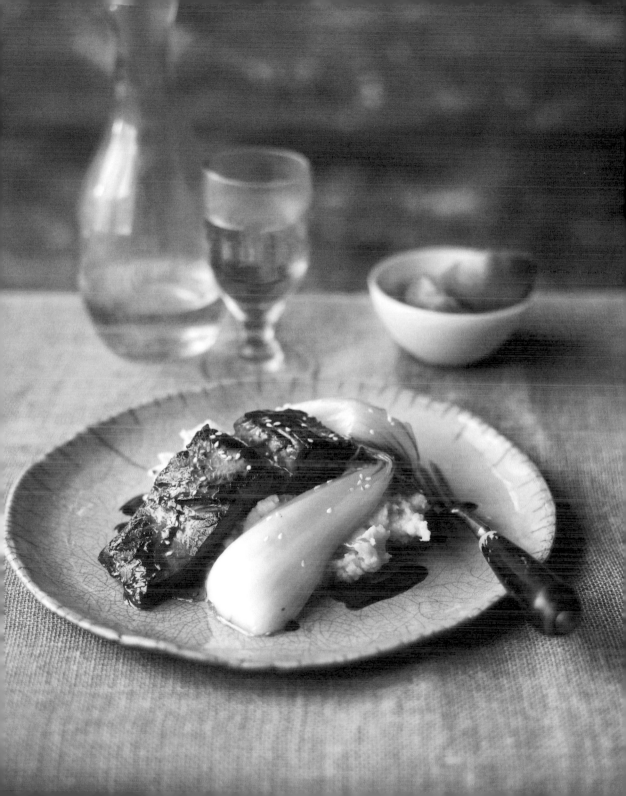

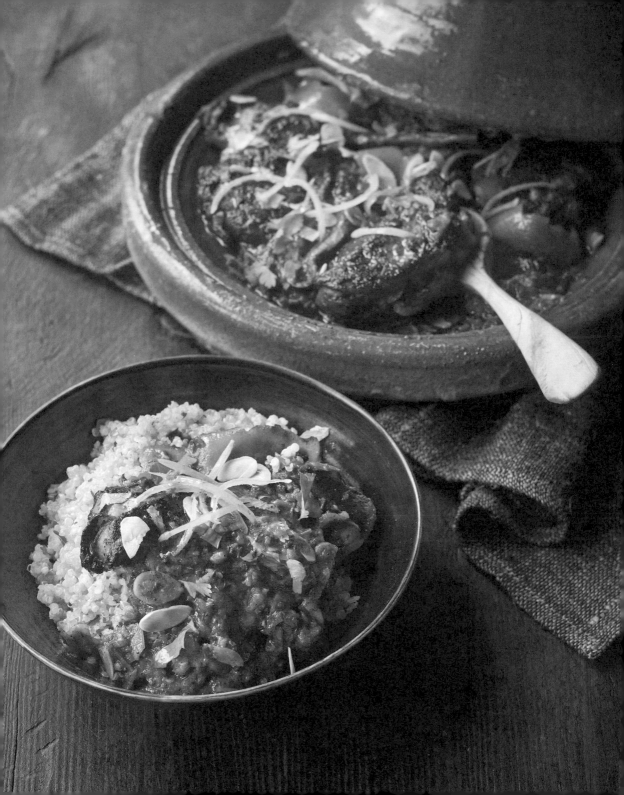

With chicken, it is often all about the flavours you put with it, which is why I love tagines — fragrant and addictive, the Persian spices and preserved lemon make for a really exotic dish. Tagines are also very healthy, full of detoxing spices and dried and fresh fruit. You can of course swap the chicken for another meat, or make a vegetarian version with some kind of squash and green vegetable. Serve it on a bed of quinoa or the vibrant red Camargue rice.

chicken tagine

2 teaspoons coriander seeds
6 chicken thighs, skin on and bone in
extra virgin olive oil
sea salt and freshly ground black pepper
good pinch of saffron threads
2 teaspoons ground cinnamon
1 teaspoon ground ginger
2 red onions, chopped
4 garlic cloves, crushed
3 tablespoons flaked/silvered almonds
2.5-cm/1-inch piece of fresh ginger, peeled and finely chopped
1 cinnamon stick
12 Medjool dates, pitted and torn into halves
1 orange, rind peeled off in strips
2 tablespoons pure maple syrup
4 tablespoons freshly chopped coriander/cilantro
1 preserved lemon
quinoa or rice, to serve

Serves 4

Put the coriander seeds in a dry pan and toast until fragrant. Pound to a powder using a pestle and mortar.

Rub the chicken thighs with a little oil, salt, pepper, the saffron threads, ground cinnamon, ginger and toasted coriander. Cover and marinate in the fridge for at least 1 hour, or you can prep them the night before.

Heat 3 tablespoons oil in a tagine or casserole dish over medium heat. Add the onions, garlic, 2 tablespoons of the almonds, the ginger, cinnamon stick and a good pinch of salt and sweat out until the onions are translucent, being careful not to burn the garlic. Transfer to a plate, and without washing the pan, add the chicken thighs. Turn up the heat to high and seal the skins, turning the chicken as it browns.

When golden brown all over, return the onion mixture to the pan. Pour in enough water to cover the chicken and bring to the boil. Reduce the heat, put the lid on and simmer for 1 hour, stirring every so often.

Add the dates, orange peel, maple syrup and half the coriander/cilantro and simmer for 20 minutes until the sauce is thick and syrupy. If you are cooking quinoa or rice, now is the time to put this on to cook.

Rinse the preserved lemon well under running water, removing as much salt as possible. Scoop out and discard the flesh, and thinly slice the skin.

Plate up the quinoa or rice with the tagine on top. Sprinkle over the preserved lemon and remaining almonds and coriander/cilantro.

Guilt-free because...

Ginger is known not only for its anti-nausea properties, but also as a potent anti-inflammatory and has demonstrated great promise in the natural treatment of arthritis. Trial participants noted less pain when they moved the affected joint and less swelling. This anti-inflammatory action appears to be due to a phenol within ginger called gingerol that stops damage from free radicals and also helps to suppress pro-inflammatory cytokines that may lead to swelling in the synovial lining of joints.

Arriving into the backpacker hive of the Kao San Road, Thailand, at the beginning of one of my first university summer holidays, I was full of expectations – not least of course, the food! I soon dove headfirst into Thai cooking in all its fiery glory. My lasting memory is of a velvety-rich, utterly addictive Massaman curry – the perfect balance of spicy, sweet and salty. It's flavourful dishes like these that make eating healthily so easy, as you don't feel deprived at all!

massaman curry

extra virgin olive oil
brown rice, to serve

Curry Paste
15 dried red chillies
1 tablespoon coriander seeds
1 teaspoon cumin seeds
1 cinnamon stick
2 cardamom pods
3 cloves
4 black peppercorns
½ teaspoon ground turmeric
1 big teaspoon shrimp paste
4 tablespoons chopped garlic
4 tablespoons chopped shallots
1–2 lemongrass sticks, chopped
2.5-cm/1 inch piece of galangal (or a smaller amount of fresh ginger), chopped
1 teaspoon nam pla fish sauce

Massaman Curry
400 ml/1⅔ cups coconut cream
4 tablespoons curry paste

600 g/1¼ oz. beef, cut into chunks
½ butternut squash, peeled, seeded and cut into chunks
200 g/7 oz. Rosevale potatoes (or other waxy potatoes), cut into chunks
1 red onion, thickly sliced
1 fresh red chilli, seeded and sliced
2 cardamom pods
1 cinnamon stick
4 kaffir lime leaves
2 tablespoons tamarind paste
2 tablespoons pure maple syrup
1 tablespoon nam pla fish sauce
2 limes – 1 juiced and the other quartered
90 g/⅔ cup cashews, lightly roasted at 180°C (350°F) Gas 4 for about 10 minutes or until they have gone a shade darker
250 g/8 oz. spinach leaves

Serves 6–8

To make the curry paste, heat the spices (apart from turmeric) in a dry frying pan over medium flame for a few minutes until fragrant. Process in a spice grinder or food processor, then if it is still very chunky, pound it to a powder using a pestle and mortar. In the same dry pan, dry fry the shrimp paste for 1 minute to bring out the flavour. In a food processor, blitz the remaining ingredients and ½ teaspoon salt. Add the spices and shrimp paste and blitz again until you have a smooth paste.

To make the massaman curry, fry 2 tablespoons of the coconut cream and all the curry paste in a large casserole dish over medium heat for 1–2 minutes until aromatic. Add the beef and fry until sealed all over. Add the remaining coconut cream, 200 ml/¾ cup water, squash, potatoes, onion, chilli (reserving some for serving), cardamom, cinnamon, lime leaves, tamarind, maple syrup, fish sauce, lime juice and the cashews (reserving some for serving). Bring to a simmer for 2 minutes, then reduce the heat to the lowest, cover with a lid and cook gently for 1 hour. (If you have loads of time, after you have brought it to simmering point you can put the entire casserole dish, with the lid on, in an oven preheated to 180°C [350°F] Gas 4 for 2 hours, until the beef is meltingly tender.)

Just before serving, add the spinach and stir until wilted. Taste and adjust the seasoning as necessary. A massaman curry needs to be quite high on salt and sweet. So, if necessary, add a little more fish sauce (or salt if you want a more neutral saltiness) and maple syrup. Serve with the remaining chilli and cashews scattered over, a drizzle of oil and the brown rice.

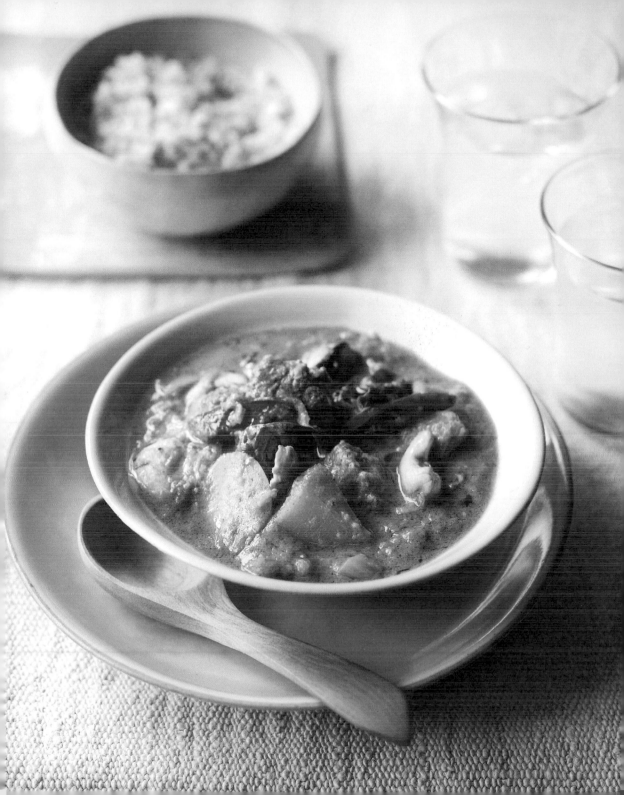

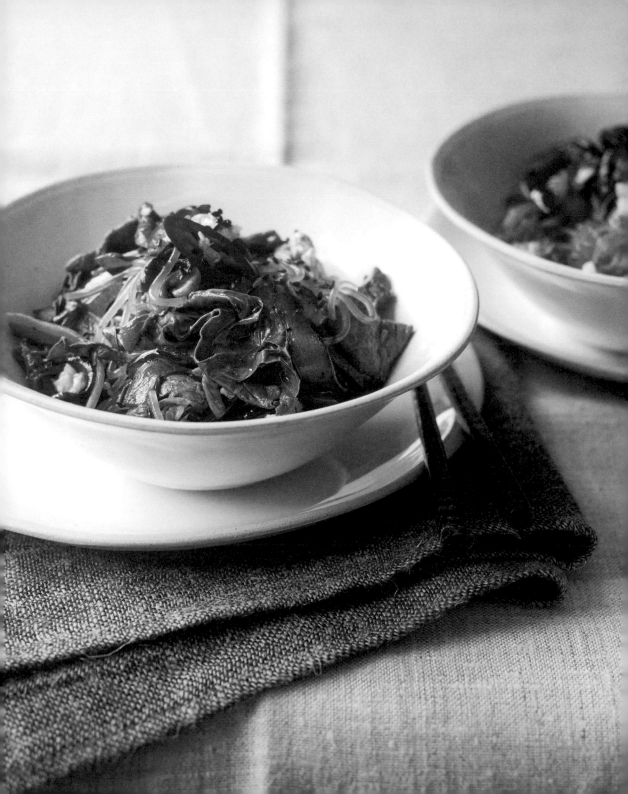

My wife Jina, who is originally from South Korea, introduced me to this dish years ago when we were travelling there, and I loved it so much that we have been making it at least once a week ever since. Not much is known about Korean food, which is a great shame as it is one of the best cuisines I have come across. Extremely healthy and full of flavour, this dish is naturally sugar, wheat and dairy free — even the noodles, which are made from sweet potatoes.

jina's jap chae with sweet potato noodles, beef, mushrooms, spinach & carrots

150 g/5 oz. beef, thinly sliced, eg. sirloin (omit if you are vegetarian)
10 shiitake mushrooms, sliced
dark soy sauce (if you have coeliac disease, use tamari soy sauce and check the label to make sure it is gluten-free)
toasted sesame oil
agave syrup
1 garlic clove, smashed
150 g/5 oz. spinach leaves
250 g/8 oz. cellophane noodles (made from sweet potato starch)
vegetable oil
100 g/3½ oz. carrot, cut into thin matchsticks
1 large red onion, sliced
1 tablespoon chilli paste (try to find authentic Korean gochujang paste in Asian stores)
1 tablespoon sesame seeds, lightly toasted
1 egg
black sesame seeds and sliced chilli, to serve
kimchi, to serve (Korean fermented cabbage)

Serves 6

Put the beef, mushrooms, 1 tablespoon soy sauce, 1 tablespoon sesame oil, 1 tablespoon agave syrup and the garlic in a bowl, make sure the beef and mushrooms are well coated and marinate for 15 minutes or a few hours if you have time.

Meanwhile, rinse the spinach, then drain and put straight into a large saucepan over high heat. Watch over it as it wilts very quickly, and stir often. Remove to a sieve/strainer and press the remaining water out of it. Put on a plate while still warm and season with a little soy sauce and sesame oil.

Cook the noodles in a large pan of boiling, salted water for 6 minutes or until tender. While they are cooking, stir-fry the beef and mushrooms with a little vegetable oil in a separate pan.

Do the same with the carrot and onions until just tender and slightly coloured, then drizzle over a little sesame oil and soy sauce.

Mix together 3 tablespoons each soy sauce and agave syrup, the chilli paste and 2½ tablespoons sesame oil.

Drain the cooked noodles well, then return to the empty pan. Add the fried vegetables, chilli sauce and sesame seeds. Crack the egg on top and, over medium heat, toss everything together until evenly mixed and the egg is cooked. It may need another dash of sesame, soy or agave depending on your tastes but don't get carried away, as they are strong flavours. Serve immediately with black sesame seeds and sliced chilli scattered over, and kimchi on the side, if you like.

Guilt-free because…

Kimchi is served by the Koreans at every meal because of its fantastic health properties. It is made by fermenting cabbage with spicy red pepper, garlic and salt. Recent studies have pointed out its anti-viral and potential anti-cancer effects, not to mention that it helps to promote healthy gut bacteria such as lactobacillus and bifidobacteria which we need for producing B vitamins and to ensure optimal immune function.

One year, on the way back to London from visiting Jina's family in Korea, we stopped off in Tokyo to sample as much authentic Japanese food as possible. Luckily, Jina had friends living there who took us to some incredible restaurants that we otherwise never would have found. The highlight was a buzzing tempura bar where pretty much anything was battered, fried and served up to you in seconds! This wheat-free version is made using rice and cornflour/cornstarch.

tempura vegetables & shrimp
with wasabi mayonnaise

selection of vegetables, eg. carrot, sweet potato, aubergine/eggplant, squash, broccoli, (bell) pepper, spring onion/scallion, beet(root)

600 ml/2½ cups vegetable, sunflower or rapeseed oil

4 king prawns/jumbo shrimp, shells and central veins removed, but tails on

100 g/¾ cup rice flour, plus extra for coating

100 g/¾ cup cornflour/cornstarch

1 teaspoon baking powder

small bottle of ice-cold sparkling water

2 egg whites

few cubes of ice

sea salt and freshly ground black pepper

Wholegrain Mustard Mayonnaise recipe (page 90), replacing the wholegrain mustard with wasabi powder or paste

Serves 4

Cut the hard vegetables into thin slices about ½ cm/¼ inch thick. Cut softer vegetables like aubergine/eggplant, spring onion/scallion or (bell) pepper a little thicker.

If you have a deep fat fryer, heat the oil to 190°C/375°F, otherwise heat it in a deep saucepan. If you don't have a cooking thermometer, check the temperature by dropping a breadcrumb into the oil. It should turn golden in about 25–30 seconds. Any faster than this and the tempura will burn before the vegetable inside is cooked through.

While the oil is heating, mix together the flours, baking powder, ½ teaspoon salt and a good pinch of pepper in a bowl. Slowly stir in just enough cold sparkling water until you have a yogurt consistency, but don't over-whisk. It doesn't matter if the batter is lumpy; traditionally Japanese tempura batter is not mixed too thoroughly, as the lumps in the batter help to form a more crunchy tempura. Using an electric whisk, beat the egg whites in a separate bowl until they form hard peaks. Fold the eggs into the batter, stir the ice cubes through to keep it as cold as possible.

Lightly coat the vegetables and prawns/shrimp in rice flour. Shake off any excess, then dip into the batter. Carefully place them into the hot oil. Don't overcrowd the fryer or pan, as it will bring down the temperature of the oil. The prawns/shrimp will take about 3 minutes and the vegetables about 2 minutes. Remove all the tempura with a slotted spoon and drain on kitchen paper/paper towels. Serve with the wasabi mayonnaise.

Guilt-free because...

The Japanese diet is widely acknowledged to be one of the healthiest in the world and a large part of that is down to the varied and regular consumption of vegetables. The Japanese consume on average 5 times as many vegetables as in the UK and this is thought to be directly linked to their slower aging and low incidence of chronic disease. Tempura is a clever way of convincing even hardcore carnivores to eat more vegetables.

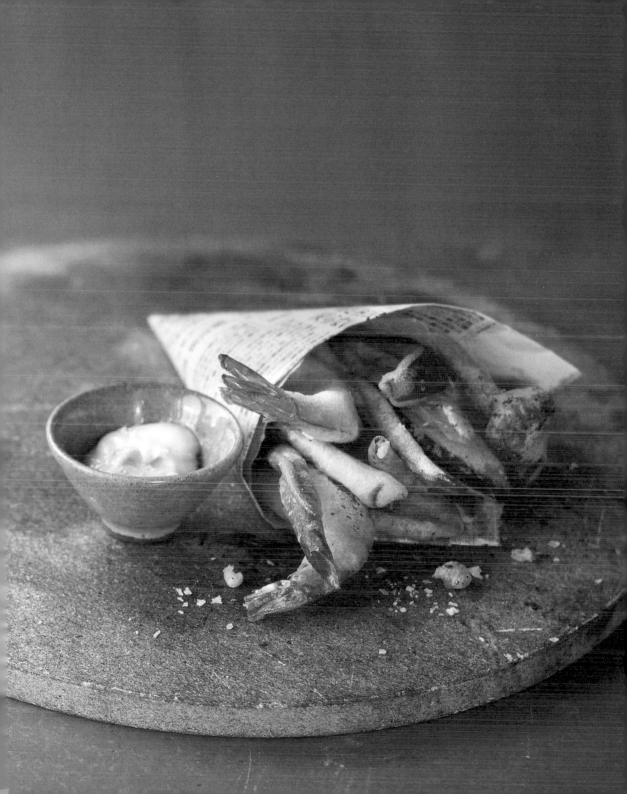

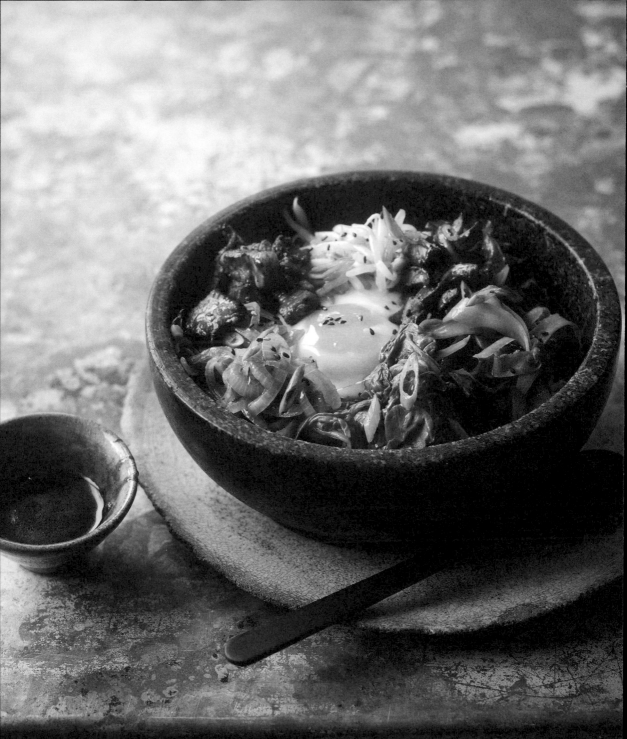

I first encountered this naturally guilt-free dish on a bitterly cold December day in Seoul, Korea. Served in a steaming hot stone bowl, the presentation was just as exciting as the punchy chilli and sesame flavours inside. Good-quality ingredients make a world of difference for a truly authentic Korean taste, and gochujang, which is a slightly sweet chilli paste, is well worth seeking out in Asian food stores.

bibimbap

400 g/14 oz. pork belly, chopped into thin 2.5-cm/1-inch pieces

400 g/2 cups short grain brown rice, eg. brown sushi rice

vegetable or sunflower oil

2 carrots, cut into thin strips

toasted sesame oil

dark soy sauce (if you have coeliac disease, use tamari soy sauce and check the label to make sure it is gluten-free)

agave syrup

150 g/5 oz. oyster or shiitake mushrooms

150 g/5 oz. bean sprouts

3 onions, sliced

200 g/6½ oz. spinach leaves

4 eggs

2 spring onions/scallions, finely chopped

black sesame seeds

Gochujang Sauce

4 tablespoons gochujang paste

4 tablespoons toasted sesame oil

4 tablespoons dark soy sauce (see above)

2 garlic cloves, crushed

1 tablespoon maple syrup

Serves 4

To make the gochujang sauce, mix together all the ingredients. Put half the sauce over the pork belly in a bowl, cover and marinate in the fridge for at least 1 hour, or more if you have time.

Cook the rice according to the packet instructions and keep warm.

While the rice is cooking, heat 1 tablespoon oil in a pan or wok and stir-fry the carrots until beginning to soften. Add ½ teaspoon sesame oil, soy sauce and maple syrup. Cook for 1 minute over high heat, then set aside on a plate. Cook the mushrooms, bean sprouts, onions, and spinach (which will wilt down) separately and in the same way, seasoning at the end. It is normal for the vegetables to be served at room temperature, as long as the rice, meat and eggs are hot, so don't worry about keeping them warm.

In the same pan you used for the vegetables, stir-fry the marinated pork (with the sauce it was sitting in) until cooked through. The sauce should reduce down a little with the heat, intensifying all the flavours.

In a separate pan, fry the 4 eggs however you like them – it is nice to have the yolk a little soft for this dish.

Serve the hot rice in 4 bowls and top with individual piles of vegetables and meat, finishing off with the egg in the middle and a sprinkling of spring onions/scallions and sesame seeds.

Serve with the remaining gochujang sauce, adding as much or as little as you like. The Korean way of eating this is to mix the whole thing together like crazy until all the ingredients are well combined. If it is not punchy enough, add more sauce.

Guilt-free because…

Shiitake mushrooms are widely renowned for their immune-promoting properties. Research has shown that they also inhibit tumour growth. Their active ingredient is a beta-glucan polysaccharide known as lentinan, which helps to activate our own immune cells so that they respond more efficiently to infection or viral growth. Please note that mushrooms of all types contain purines which may be problematic for those with excess uric acid build-up, e.g. gout and kidney stones.

comfort food

I grew up in Ireland where the rain and cold are your long-time companions, so comfort foods play a very important part in daily life! Here is a selection of truly indulgent recipes that are as creamy and comforting as you could possibly hope for, yet without any of the guilt. So go on, close the curtains, curl up on the sofa and warm up with one of these cosy dishes.

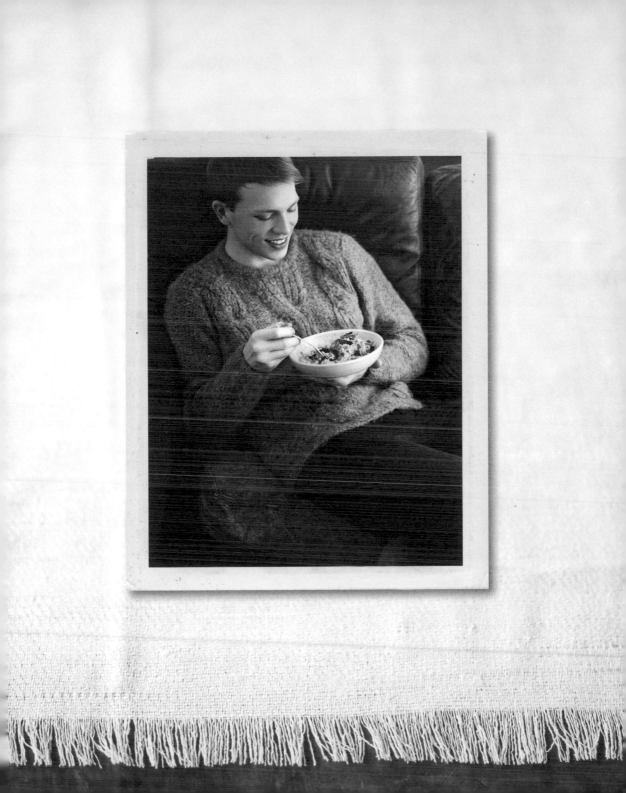

handful of fresh dill
handful of fresh parsley
leaves from 2 sprigs fresh
   thyme
350 g/11 oz. beet(root),
   grated
150 g/5 oz. carrot, finely
   grated
120 g/1 cup oatmeal
3 eggs
1 small red onion, finely
   chopped
2 garlic cloves, crushed
sea salt and freshly
   ground black pepper
1 tablespoon vegetable oil
wheat-free bread rolls
rocket/arugula
cherry tomatoes, halved

Wholegrain Mustard
Mayonnaise
300 ml/1¼ cups good
   extra virgin olive oil
300 ml/1¼ cups
   sunflower oil
2 egg yolks
1 teaspoon Dijon mustard
squeeze of lemon juice
3 teaspoons wholegrain
   mustard

Slaw
½ small celeriac/celery
   root, cut into thin
   matchsticks
½ red cabbage, very thinly
   sliced
2 carrots, shredded
1 red onion, thinly sliced
small handful of hazelnuts,
   toasted and chopped
3 tablespoons freshly
   chopped parsley
2 eating apples
grated zest of 1 lemon,
   plus juice of ½

Makes about 10

There is no question that reducing the amount of meat in your diet is not only good for your health but also for the planet. So before you go running for the hills at the mention of a 'veggie' burger, at least taste this one before you make any judgments. It is not an attempt to replicate a beef burger but it is very similar in texture, just as satisfying, and has gone down really well with my carnivore friends.

beetroot burgers with wholegrain mustard mayonnaise

Finely chop the herbs. Thoroughly combine with the beet(root), carrot, oatmeal, eggs, onion and garlic in a bowl, making sure the eggs and herbs are evenly distributed. Season with 1 teaspoon salt and a few grindings of pepper. Set aside for 15 minutes.

To make the wholegrain mustard mayonnaise, you can use a food processor or an electric whisk. Either way, combine the oils in a jug. Put the egg yolks, Dijon mustard, lemon juice and a pinch of salt in the food processor bowl or a mixing bowl. As you start to process/whisk, very slowly feed in the oils a little at a time until the mixture begins to emulsify and come together. Once this happens you can add the oil a bit faster, but never be tempted to fire it all in otherwise the mayonnaise will split. I always have a little cup of boiling water ready, as a few drops added in when it is looking like it might split usually brings it back together. Once you have added all the oil, stir in the wholegrain mustard and refrigerate until needed.

To make the slaw, combine the celeriac/celery root, cabbage, carrots, onion, hazelnuts and most of the parsley in a bowl. When you are ready to serve the slaw, cut the apple into thin half-moon slices, getting rid of the core, and mix into the bowl. Add 3 tablespoons of the wholegrain mustard mayonnaise, 1 tablespoon oil, the lemon zest and juice, ½ teaspoon salt and a pinch of pepper and mix well with your hands. Taste and if necessary, add a little extra salt, olive oil or wholegrain mustard.

Preheat the oven to 180°C (350°F) Gas 4.

To make the burgers, form about 10 patties with your hands. Heat the vegetable oil in a frying pan over low heat and fry the burgers until just browned – 2–3 minutes on each side. Transfer to an ovenproof dish and bake in the preheated oven for 20 minutes.

Toast the bread rolls or pita bread, if you like. Cut them open and spread the wholegrain mustard mayonnaise on the inside. Add the rocket/arugula, some halved tomatoes, some slaw and a burger.

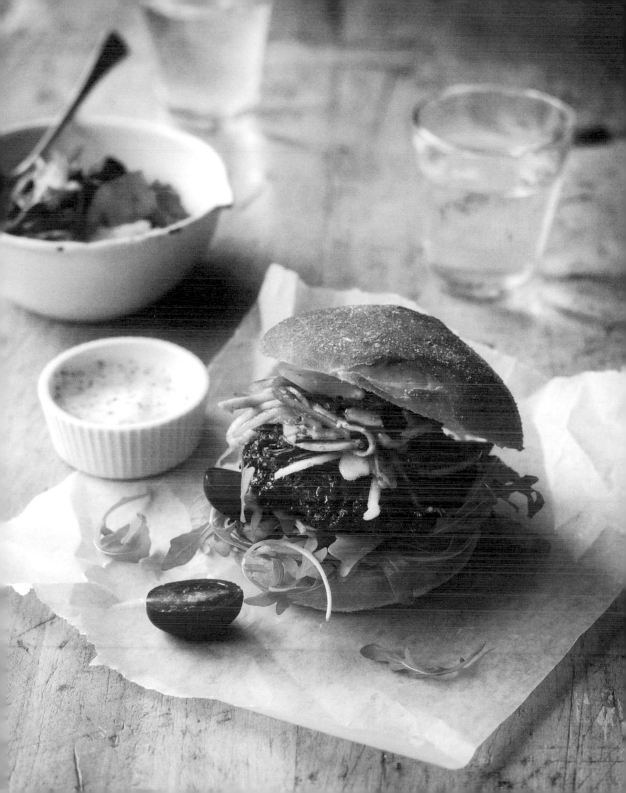

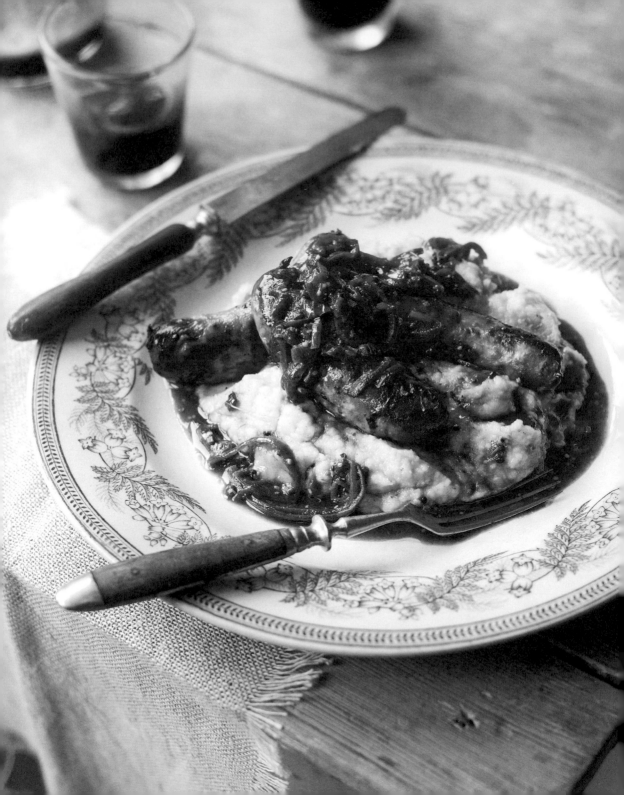

Who doesn't love sausages 'n' mash? I am actually having great difficulty writing this introduction without giving into the urge to run off and make this dish immediately. It really is the ultimate in comfort food and when served with a really good onion gravy and wholegrain mustard, this can be a stellar dish. I am using butter beans for the mash, which work incredibly well.

sausages 'n' mash with red onion gravy

extra virgin olive oil
2 red onions, sliced
1 tablespoon fresh rosemary needles, chopped
5 garlic cloves, chopped
2 tablespoons balsamic vinegar
1 teaspoon agave syrup
1 teaspoon bouillon stock powder or ½ cube, dissolved in 300 ml/ 1¼ cups water
2 teaspoons wholegrain mustard
sea salt
2 x 400-g/14-oz. cans butter beans
1 teaspoon fresh thyme leaves
2 teaspoons Dijon mustard
grated zest of ½ lemon
4–6 sausages (made with at least 85% meat; look for wheat-free sausages made without breadcrumbs if you like, or even vegetarian ones)

Serves 2–3

Start off with the gravy. Gently sweat the onions, rosemary and 2 of the chopped garlic cloves in a little oil in a saucepan for about 15 minutes or until the onions are soft and translucent. Add the vinegar and agave syrup and continue to cook over slightly higher heat for another 15 minutes. You want the onions to caramelize a little, but be careful not to burn them. Add the stock and wholegrain mustard, bring to the boil, then turn the heat down and cook until the gravy has reduced. Taste and adjust the seasoning.

Drain the butter beans and warm in a pan with some oil, the rest of the garlic and the thyme. This will only take a few minutes – you do not want to colour the garlic at all, just heat it through and release its flavour. Throw this all into a food processor, add the Dijon mustard, a few glugs of oil, the lemon zest and a good pinch of salt. Blend until smooth; you will most likely need another bit of oil (depending on the consistency you want). Add more mustard and salt if it needs it, as the butter beans soak up a lot of flavour.

Fry or grill/broil the sausages, then dollop the butter-bean mash onto the middle of a plates, nestle the sausages on top and pour over as much of the onion gravy as you like. Serve with some more wholegrain mustard.

Guilt-free because...

Butter beans are a useful source of fibre, magnesium and folate, which are nutrients known to reduce cholesterol and improve heart health. They are also extremely high in a lesser known micro-mineral called molybdenum. It works with copper to control how iron is moved and released within the body, which is an important action as without it our tissue oxygen needs will not be met. A 200-g/7-oz. serving of butter beans will provide you with over 80% of your daily requirement of molybdenum.

Lasagna was at the height of its fame in the 80s and early 90s but its warming and creamy texture has made sure its popularity has not waned too much since. It is perfect for weekend cooking, as it does take a bit of time. Making a wheat-free béchamel sauce is also really simple using rice flour and it tastes precisely the same.

lasagna

sea salt and freshly
    ground black pepper
extra virgin olive oil
1 large onion, finely
    chopped
1 carrot, finely chopped
2 celery sticks, finely
    chopped
6 garlic cloves, crushed
500 g/1 lb. minced/
    ground beef (lean
    is best)
50 g/1½ oz. pancetta,
    chopped
sprig fresh thyme
sprig fresh rosemary
2 dried bay leaves
200 ml/¾ cup red wine

2 x 400-g/14-oz. cans
    chopped tomatoes
    (the best you can find)
½ teaspoon grated
    nutmeg
10–12 gluten-free pasta
    sheets
4 tablespoons spelt or
    wheat-free breadcrumbs
    mixed with 1
    tablespoon mixed
    herbs, eg. thyme,
    rosemary and parsley,
    and a pinch of salt and
    pepper

Béchamel Sauce
600 ml/2½ cups rice milk
½ carrot, sliced
½ onion, sliced
4 black peppercorns
1 clove
2 dried bay leaves
sprig fresh thyme
a few stalks fresh parsley
50 ml/3 tablespoons
    olive oil
50 g/6 tablespoons
    gluten-free flour, or
    25 g/3 tablespoons
    each rice flour and
    cornflour/cornstarch

20-cm/8-inch-long
    rectangular lasagna
    dish, greased

Serves 6

To make the béchamel sauce, put the milk, carrot, onion, peppercorns, clove, bay leaves and herbs in a saucepan and bring to the boil. Simmer for a few minutes, then remove from the heat and allow to cool. When cool, strain. Gently warm the oil in a pan. Slowly add the flour, stirring until incorporated, then whisk in the infused milk, a little at a time, until thick. Season with a pinch of salt.

Heat 1 tablespoon oil in a large, heavy-bottomed casserole dish over medium heat. Add the onions and cook until translucent but not coloured. Add the carrot, celery and a good pinch of salt and sweat down gently for another few minutes. Add the garlic and cook for 1–2 minutes until the flavour is released. Add the beef, pancetta, herbs and bay leaves and stir, breaking up the beef. Cook over low–medium heat until cooked through but not coloured. Season to taste with salt and pepper. Add the wine, bring to the boil and cook until evaporated. Add the tomato and nutmeg, bring to the boil and cook for 10 minutes. Reduce the heat to the lowest setting and cook very gently, uncovered, for 1½ hours, stirring occasionally. If the sauce becomes too thick, add a little water. Season to taste with salt and pepper.

Preheat the oven to 220°C (425°F) Gas 7.

Spread some of the béchamel over the base of the lasagna dish. Cover with pasta sheets, breaking them where necessary. Spread some meat sauce on top, then a layer of béchamel. Cover with pasta sheets and continue like this until you are ¼ cm/½ inch below the top. Finish with a layer of pasta coated with béchamel, then sprinkle over the breadcrumb mixture. Cook in the preheated oven for 30 minutes or until the pasta is cooked through and the top is golden brown. Allow to rest for 15 minutes before serving.

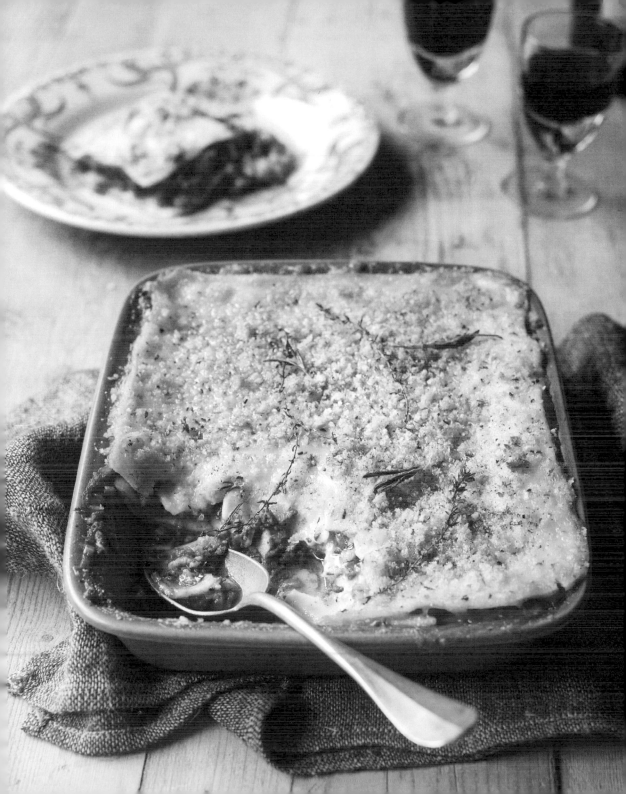

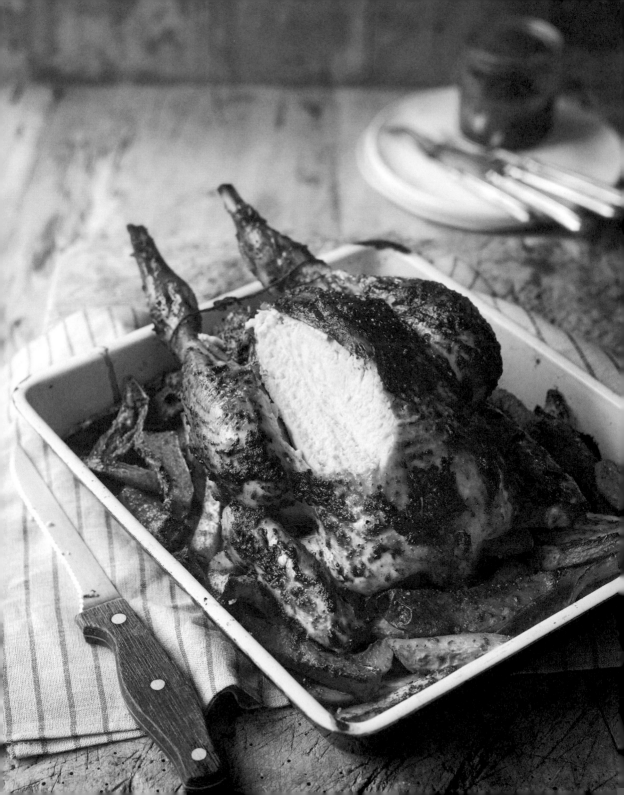

I love roast chicken for all the memories and images that it brings to mind when I cook it — my family home, the smell, a tableful of people, my mother and non-stop chatter. For me, food is so much more than mere sustenance — it's about the way it makes you feel and how it can bring people together. This is the perfect dish for a relaxed meal with friends and family: minimum fuss but maximum taste.

harissa roast chicken
with spiced swede, squash & sweet potato

extra virgin olive oil
2 teaspoons cumin seeds
2 teaspoons coriander seeds
1 swede/rutabaga, peeled and chopped into chunks
1 butternut squash, peeled, seeded and chopped into chunks
2 sweet potatoes, chopped into chunks
2 teaspoons ground turmeric
sea salt
2 tablespoons soy yogurt
1 free-range, organic chicken
1 lemon
green salad, to serve

Harissa Paste
2 teaspoons each cumin, coriander and caraway seeds
1 red onion, chopped
3 garlic cloves, chopped
2–3 red chillies, seeded
4 jarred Piquillo peppers
3 teaspoons tomato purée/concentrate
2 tablespoons lemon juice
1 teaspoon sweet smoked paprika

To make the harissa paste, put the cumin, coriander and caraway seeds in a dry pan and toast for 1–2 minutes until you can smell the aromas wafting up from the pan. Pound to a powder using a pestle and mortar. In the same pan, heat a little oil and very gently fry the onion, garlic and chillies until all soft. Transfer, with the Piquillo peppers, tomato purée/concentrate, lemon juice, paprika, 4 tablespoons oil and a pinch of salt, to a food processor and process until smooth. You may need to adjust the seasoning slightly with a little more salt, paprika or lemon juice.

Preheat the oven to 240°C (475°F) Gas 9.

For the vegetables, toast and grind the cumin and coriander seeds as above. In a bowl, toss the chopped vegetables with 1 teaspoon salt, all the spices and enough oil to coat them generously. Transfer to a roasting pan, making sure to get all the oil and spices out of the bowl and onto the vegetables.

Mix together 3 tablespoons of your harissa paste with the yogurt. Season the chicken with salt and pepper, then spread the harissa mixture all over the skin, pushing some underneath the skin

as well. Add some more harissa paste if you want it more spicy. Prick the lemon all over with a sharp knife and place inside the cavity of the chicken.

Place the chicken directly on top of the vegetables and place in the middle of the oven. Immediately turn the heat down to 180°C (350°F) Gas 4 and roast for 30 minutes or until the chicken is beginning to brown.

Remove the roasting pan from the oven, lift the chicken onto a board and stir the vegetables well to make sure they're completely coated in all the juices. Return the chicken to the roasting pan, baste the breast with the juices and continue to roast for a further 40–50 minutes until cooked all the way through; you can check this by inserting a skewer into the leg and if the juices run clear, it is cooked. If the skin looks like it is going to burn at any stage, cover with foil. You do want the skin to be nice and crispy though, so don't cover it in anticipation of burning.

Once the chicken is cooked, wrap the tray in foil for 15 minutes before serving — this allows the flesh to relax and become more tender. Serve with a big green salad.

Serves 6–8

I can't tell you how comforting this soup is. The sweet smoked paprika and the gentle heat from the chilli warm up even the most wind-swept and bitterly cold winter days. The root vegetable crisps/chips work very well with it, adding a lovely and satisfying crunch. Try and get the Spanish brands of sweet smoked paprika that come in little tins, as they have excellent flavour.

red pepper & smoked paprika soup
with basil oil & vegetable crisps

300 g/10 oz. baby plum tomatoes – as ripe and red as you can find
extra virgin olive oil
sea salt and freshly ground black pepper
2 red onions, chopped
2 red chillies, seeded and finely chopped
3 garlic cloves, finely chopped
4 red (bell) peppers, seeded and chopped
1 sweet potato, peeled and chopped into cubes
700 ml/3 cups vegetable stock/broth
2 teaspoons sweet smoked paprika
8–10 fresh basil leaves
vegetable crisps/chips (you can get these in good supermarkets and any root vegetable will do, eg. parsnip, sweet potato or beet[root])

Serves 6–8

Preheat the oven to 180°C (350°F) Gas 4.

Toss the tomatoes in a little oil and salt on a baking sheet. Roast in the preheated oven for about 15 minutes, or until they have shrivelled up a bit and the skins have popped open.

Heat 3 tablespoons of oil in a heavy-based saucepan over low heat, add the onions, chillies and garlic and sweat out until the onions are translucent. Add 2 pinches of salt. Add the (bell) peppers and potato and cook over low–medium heat for a further 20 minutes or until the vegetables have softened.

Add the roasted tomatoes and all the juices and the vegetable stock/broth. Bring to the boil and simmer for 10 minutes or until all the vegetables are completely soft. Using a food processor or blender, liquidize the soup until smooth. Return to the pan and add the paprika. Season to taste – it will need more salt and some pepper.

Finely chop the basil and mix together with 4 tablespoons olive oil. Ladle the soup into bowls, then with a teaspoon swirl some of the basil oil over the top and lightly place a few vegetable crisps/chips in the middle of the soup. Serve immediately.

Guilt-free because…

Red (bell) peppers are high in a number of important antioxidants. It is the combination of vitamins C, E and the carotenoids (alpha-carotene, beta-carotene, lycopene, lutein and zeaxanthin) that ensure they pack a strong nutritious punch. Zeaxanthin is found in high levels in the retina of the eye, which means red (bell) peppers should form part of any diet used to help those with macular degeneration. Lutein and zeaxanthin are also known to improve the elasticity of the skin as well as a reduction in skin lipid oxidation, a common cause of skin aging.

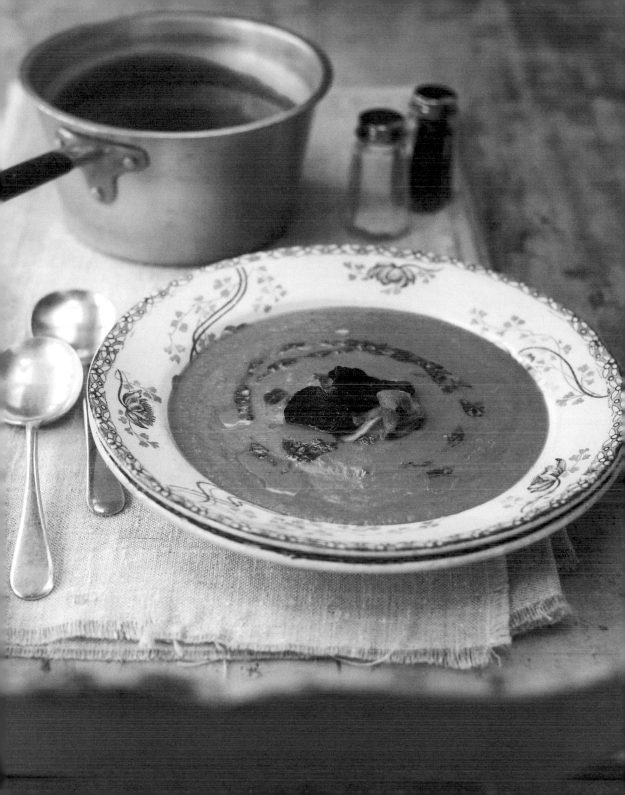

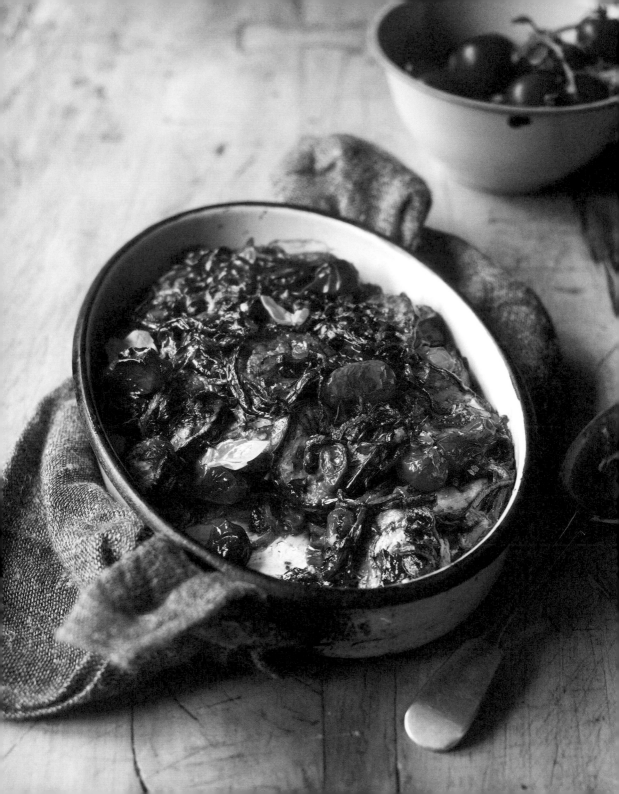

The velvety creaminess of this dish just screams 'bad for you', so it is such a joy to be able to scream back 'no it's not!' Aubergine/eggplant can be quite bland if not really encouraged with good seasoning, so this is the perfect dish for them — the tomatoes, oil, non-dairy cream and herbs really bring it to life.

aubergine & tomato gratin

2 red onions, sliced
10 cherry tomatoes –
    as ripe and red as you
    can find
extra virgin olive oil
sea salt and freshly
    ground black pepper
balsamic vinegar
3 aubergines/eggplants,
    topped, tailed and cut
    into 1-cm/½-inch slices
handful of fresh basil
    leaves
100 ml/6 tablespoons
    soy cream/creamer

Serves 4–6

Preheat the oven to 200°C (400°F) Gas 6.

Toss the onions and tomatoes with some oil, salt and a drizzle of balsamic vinegar in an ovenproof dish. Roast in the preheated oven for about 15 minutes or until the skins of the tomatoes crack open and the onions are beginning to caramelize. Leave the oven on.

Meanwhile, heat a saucepan over medium heat. Using a pastry brush, coat the aubergine/eggplant slices with oil on both sides. Fry in the hot pan until golden brown on both sides and beginning to get soft. Transfer to a dish and give them a generous drizzle of oil. Season well with salt and a little pepper.

Layer the aubergine/eggplant slices in a casserole dish with the tomatoes, onions and basil leaves (reserving some for serving). Pour the cream over, drizzle over some oil and bake in the oven for 15–20 minutes until bubbling and golden on top.

Remove from the oven. Tear the remaining basil leaves and scatter over the top of the dish. Serve immediately

Guilt-free because…

Tomatoes contain a carotenoid called lycopene, which has demonstrated anti-cancer properties. A study of men in America who consumed at least 4 servings per week of tomato products showed a 40% reduction in risk of developing prostate cancer and in newly diagnosed cases, a significant decrease in cancer progression was seen in those regularly eating tomatoes. Cooking tomatoes greatly increases the bio-availability of lycopene and the addition of olive oil further increases absorption rates of this super nutrient.

It's nice to think that a dish you associate with butter, cream and Parmesan can be just as enjoyable and indulgent when made with a few healthier alternatives. I use soy cream/creamer to give it that velvety smoothness. It has the same consistency as normal cream, and the slight difference in taste is undetectable in the risotto when seasoned properly. If you can find them in a farmers' market, buy the amazing 'trompettes de la mort' mushrooms (trumpets of death).

wild mushroom & leek risotto

900 ml/3¾ cups vegetable stock/broth (make your own by covering carrots, onion, celery, bay leaf, parsley, thyme and a few peppercorns with water and simmering for ½ hour)

extra virgin olive oil

1 large onion, finely chopped

2 leeks, chopped

6 garlic cloves, finely chopped

350 g/1¾ cups Arborio or Carnaroli rice

glass of dry white wine (if you are trying to avoid alcohol sugar, this cooks off during cooking)

sea salt and freshly ground black pepper

200 ml/¾ cup soy cream/creamer

300 g/10 oz. mixed wild mushrooms

3 tablespoons finely chopped parsley

Serves 6–8

Bring and keep the vegetable stock/broth in a saucepan just under boiling point, ready to add into the risotto.

Heat 3 tablespoons oil in a heavy-based pan, add the onion and leeks and cook gently over low heat until they are completely soft and translucent. You do not want to colour them. Add 5 of the chopped garlic cloves, turn up the heat and stir for 1 minute. Add the rice, stirring frequently until the grains are completely covered in oil and beginning to turn translucent.

Pour in the glass of wine (it should steam and bubble) and season with a pinch of salt. Gradually add the hot stock a ladleful at a time, adding another ladle each time the liquid has been absorbed by the rice.

When the stock is finished, stir through the soy cream/creamer and some pepper. Season to taste, then turn down the heat.

In a separate pan, warm a little oil over medium–high heat. Add the mushrooms and fry for 1–2 minutes until the mushrooms have softened and coloured a little.

Add the mushrooms to the risotto. Make a quick parsley oil by combining the chopped parsley with the remaining chopped garlic clove and as much oil as you like. Drizzle over the risotto and serve immediately.

Guilt-free because…

Leeks form part of the allium family of vegetables that also includes garlic and onions. This trio are collectively known for their heart health-promoting, anti-inflammatory properties. In particular, leeks have a high concentration of a flavonoid called kaempferol, which protects the blood vessels from free-radical damage. It achieves this by increasing the production of nitric oxide, which helps to relax and dilate the blood vessels, thereby reducing the likelihood of blood clots occurring. High levels of the polyphenol gallic acid also assist in the protection of the blood vessels.

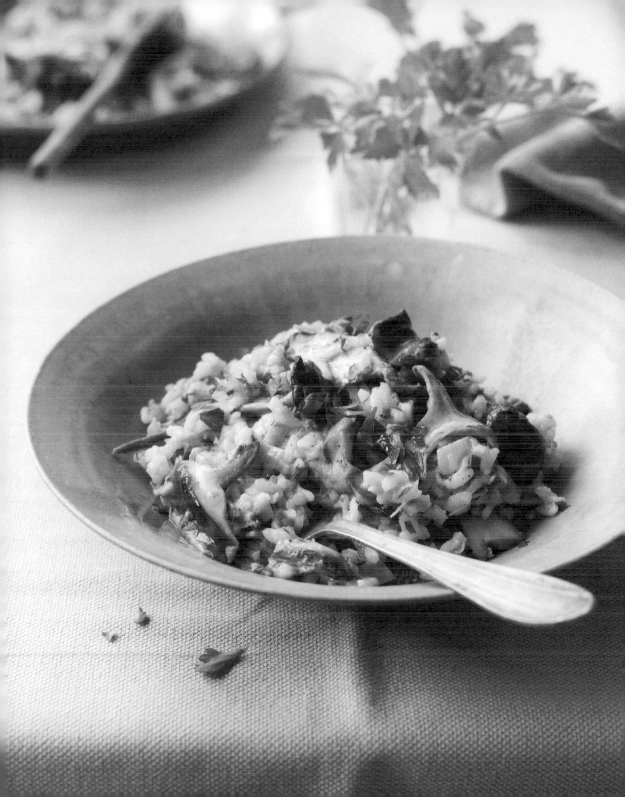

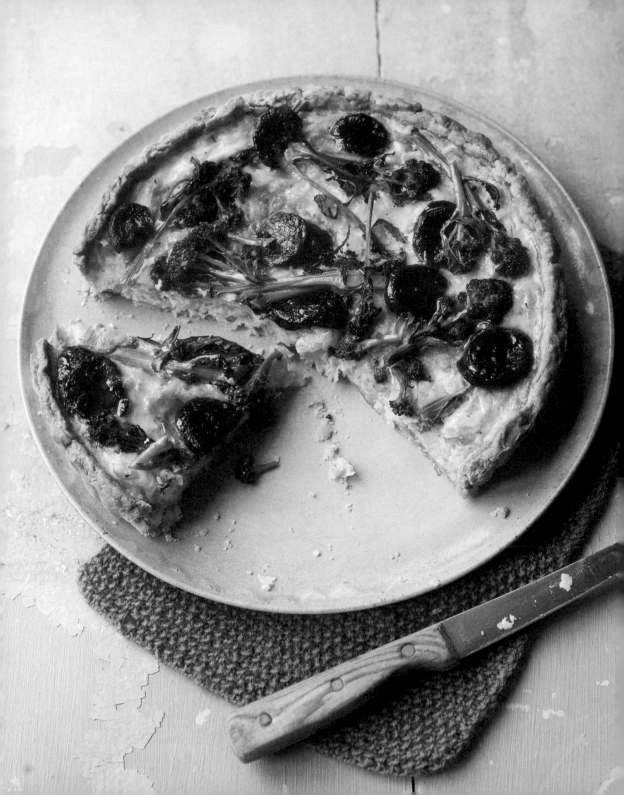

It is often the simplest and most comforting dishes that seem to achieve cult status, and tarts are definitely one of them. Whether it is the never-ending possibilities for fillings or the cosy and comforting baking smell that you get when cooking them, there are few who would turn down the offer of a slice. Using healthier alternatives for the wheat and dairy, I have often served this for lunch or dinner without anyone realizing it was any different to the average tart.

leek, sprouting broccoli & chorizo tart

Pastry
225 g/1¾ cups white spelt flour (for a wheat- and gluten-free alternative, see page 124)
pinch of sea salt
50 g/3 tablespoons dairy-free butter, e.g. sunflower spread
60 g/¼ cup hard white vegetable shortening (it is crucial that you get the hardest one you can find)
1 egg, beaten together with 1 teaspoon water

Filling
3 leeks, finely chopped
1 onion, sliced
3 garlic cloves, crushed
sea salt and freshly ground black pepper
10 spears of sprouting broccoli
100 g/3½ oz. good chorizo, skinned and chopped (omit if you are vegetarian)
3 eggs
100 ml/6 tablespoons soy cream/creamer
extra virgin olive oil

20-cm/8-inch tart pan
baking beans

Serves 8–10

To make the pastry, follow the method for the Lemon Tart on page 124 (omitting the xylitol) until you have blind-baked the tart and taken it out to cool.

To make the filling, heat 3 tablespoons oil in a large saucepan over medium heat. Add the leeks, onion, garlic and a good pinch of salt and pepper and sweat out until completely soft and translucent. About 10 minutes before they are done, trim the bases off the broccoli spears and add them in.

Heat another pan over medium heat. Add the chorizo to the dry pan and cook until a little crispy and the fat has seeped out. Add to the leek and broccoli mixture and combine. Season to taste – it should be a little saltier than you think, as the cream and egg will water it down a little.

Preheat the oven to 200°C (400°F) Gas 6.

Add the cooked mixture to the blind-baked tart shell, reserving a little of the mixture for the top of the tart. Beat the eggs together with the cream and pour into the tart shell. Scatter the reserved ingredients over the top so they are completely visible, as this makes the tart much more attractive when it is cooked.

Bake the tart in the preheated oven until the top has browned a little and is firm – 30–35 minutes or so depending on your oven. Remove from the oven and serve immediately with olive oil drizzled over.

Guilt-free because...

Broccoli has had, to date, more than 300 research trials conducted with it to understand whether it could have a beneficial impact on cancer. The results indicate that components found within it are involved in 3 key areas of cancer incidence: inflammation, oxidative stress and detoxification.

This is the ultimate comfort food — fast, filling and packed full of flavour. I have used roasted cashews instead of pine nuts in this pesto as I think they work exceptionally well with the basil, and give a really satisfying, chewy texture to the dish.

pasta with cashew pesto
& roasted cherry tomatoes

60 g/½ cup cashews
15 cherry tomatoes
extra virgin olive oil
sea salt
400 g/14 oz. brown rice
   pasta or maize pasta
   (preferably fusilli)
3 big handfuls of fresh
   basil

Serves 4–6

Preheat the oven to 200°C (400°F) Gas 6.

Spread the cashews out on a baking sheet and roast in the preheated oven until golden. Watch like a hawk as they go from just under to burned to a cinder in seconds. Leave the oven on.

Toss the tomatoes, 1 tablespoon oil and some salt on a baking sheet. Roast in the oven until the skins pop open.

Bring a large saucepan of water to the boil, add the pasta and cook until just done. As with any pasta, use a large pan with plenty of water and give it lots of room to move around. Otherwise it ends up sticking together in one big starchy mass.

Meanwhile, blitz the roasted cashews in a food processor until they are the consistency of breadcrumbs. Add the basil leaves (reserving some for serving) and pulse until well combined. Add a good pinch or 2 of salt (it takes quite a bit) and drizzle in oil until you reach your desired consistency. I like mine quite loose, but it is up to you. The key to a great pesto is in the extra virgin olive oil. Buy the best you can afford, as the depth of flavour varies greatly from oil to oil.

Drain the cooked pasta, keeping a small amount of the cooking liquid. Put the pasta back into the cooking pan, add the pesto and gently combine. If you want a bit more of a sauce, add a little of the cooking liquid and/or oil.

Finally, add the tomatoes and reserved basil leaves. Serve immediately in a large bowl, but not before you get into your pajamas so you are ready to cosy onto the sofa!

Guilt-free because…

Cashews have less fat than other nuts and the majority is in the form of oleic acid, the same heart-healthy fat found in olive oil. They are high in magnesium, which helps with cramps, as it helps muscles to relax. Cashews have been shown to reduce the risk of developing colon cancer, thought to be due to high levels of proanthocyanidins which starve tumours and prevent cancer cell division.

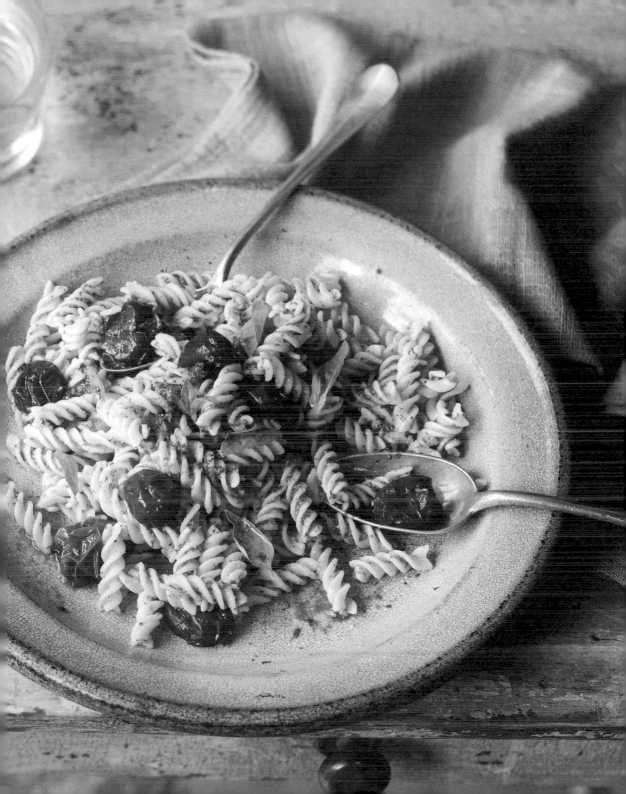

home baking

Who doesn't love the comforting, sweet smell of a cake baking in the oven? From flapjacks and brownies to fruit crumbles and muffins, there is something about home-baked goods that makes everything seem right with the world. Using natural and healthy alternatives to sugar, wheat and dairy, you can now luxuriate in these heavenly yet sin-free treats.

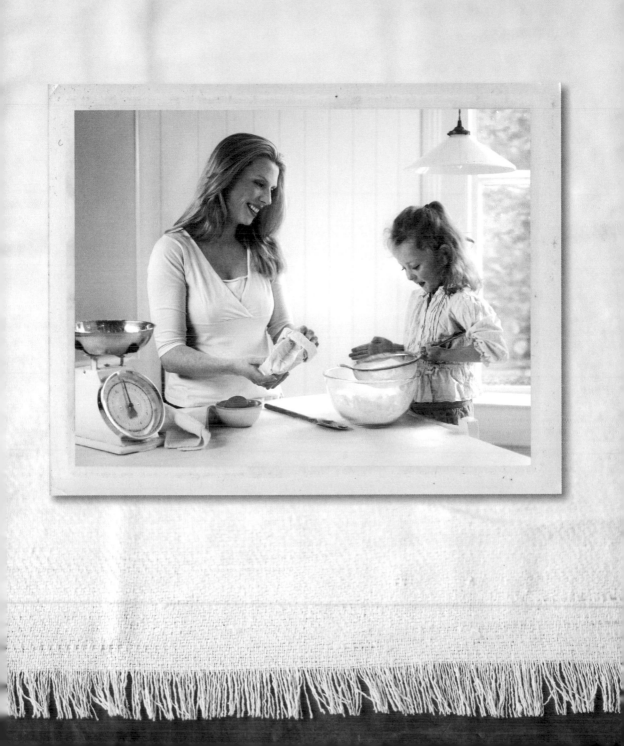

When I lived in New York, a friend of mine took me to a café called Alice's Tea Cup to try what he described as 'insanely good carrot cake'… and indeed it was. However, my sister then managed to come up with this guilt-free carrot cake, which I think knocks the socks off its New York rival. Luxuriously moist and dense with the perfect creamy topping, no one ever believes it is sugar, wheat and dairy free.

jessica's carrot cake

270 g/2 cups plus 2 tablespoons rice flour (if you can handle gluten, you can also use white spelt flour)
2 teaspoons bicarbonate of/baking soda
1 teaspoon baking powder
¼ teaspoon sea salt
2 teaspoons ground cinnamon
2 teaspoons mixed/apple pie spice
3 eggs
200 ml/1 cup rice milk
1 tablespoon lemon juice
200 ml/¾ cup vegetable, rapeseed, grapeseed or sunflower oil
280 g/1½ cups xylitol

2 teaspoons pure vanilla extract
230 g/1 generous cup grated carrots
200 g/2 cups desiccated coconut, plus extra to dust
60 g/½ cup walnuts, fresh from the shell
227-g/8-oz. can natural pineapple in juice, finely chopped
120 g/1 scant cup raisins

Frosting
227-g/8-oz. container Tofutti Cream Cheese
2 tablespoons agave syrup
grated zest of 2 lemons

2 x 20-cm/8-inch cake pans, lined with parchment paper

Serves 10—12

Preheat the oven to 180°C (350°F) Gas 4.

In a bowl, sift together the flour, bicarbonate of/baking soda, baking powder, salt, cinnamon and mixed/apple pie spice. In another bowl, combine the eggs, milk, lemon juice, oil, xylitol and vanilla extract and mix well. Add the dry ingredients and mix well.

In another bowl, combine the carrots, coconut, walnuts, pineapple and raisins. Using a large wooden spoon or in a food mixer, add this to the cake mixture and combine very well. Pour the cake mixture into the prepared cake pans and bake in the preheated oven for 1 hour or until a skewer inserted in the middle come out just clean. If it doesn't, cover the cake with foil (so it does not burn) and bake for another 10 minutes or until the skewer comes out clean. Allow to cool completely, then turn out onto a wire rack.

To make the frosting, combine all the ingredients. Spread half the frosting over one cool cake, then place the other cake on top and spread the remaining frosting over the top. To serve, liberally sprinkle desiccated coconut over the frosting.

Guilt-free because…

Carrot is popularly believed to stop us going 'blind'. This is virtually true because the eye's retina needs vitamin A to function properly. Carrots are very rich in beta-carotene which the body converts into vitamin A in the liver. Studies have also isolated a component in carrots called falcarinol which has demonstrated anti-cancer effects. Further research states that those who consume more than 6 carrots a week versus those who only ate 1 carrot a month, were much less likely to suffer a stroke.

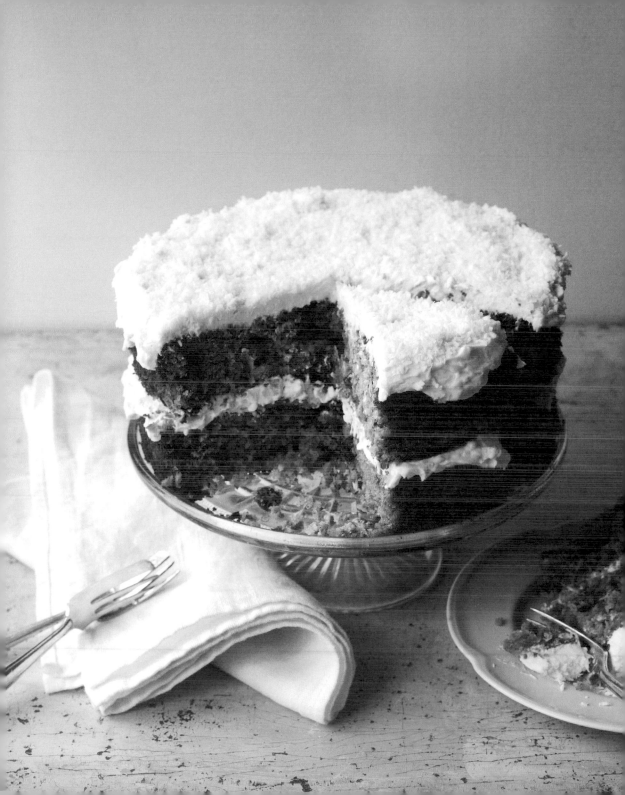

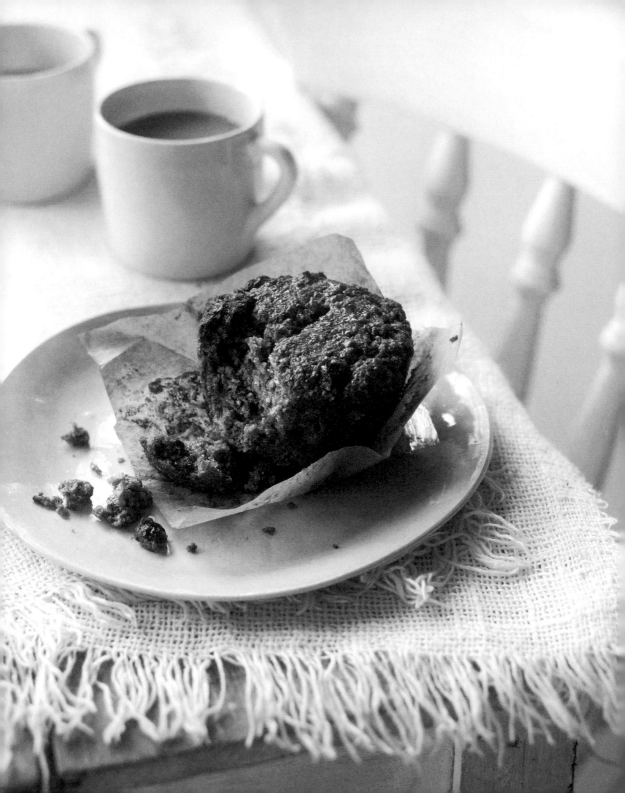

More like mini cakes than muffins, the spelt flour gives these a wonderfully chewy texture and the apples keep them nice and moist, so they taste just as good the next day… although if you are anything like me, you will have them all polished off in one sitting. These are great for breakfast, or to bring to work for an indulgent yet healthy snack. If you are coeliac, you can use rice flour.

apple, raisin & cinnamon muffins

1 cooking apple, peeled, cored and diced
150 g/1 cup plus 2 tablespoons spelt flour
150 g/1¼ cups rolled oats
100 g/⅔ cup raisins
2 teaspoons baking powder
1 teaspoon bicarbonate of/baking soda
3 teaspoons ground cinnamon
1 teaspoon mixed/ apple pie spice
¼ teaspoon grated nutmeg
good pinch of sea salt
2 eggs, lightly beaten
125 ml/½ cup soy yogurt
220 ml/1 scant cup pure maple syrup
1 eating apple, peeled, cored and diced

muffin pan (see method)

Makes 6 large muffins

Preheat the oven to 180°C (350°F) Gas 4.

Grease the muffin pan, or line it with muffin cases, or make your own muffin cases with squares of parchment paper pushed into the muffin holes.

Put the chopped cooking apple in a small saucepan with 3 tablespoons water. Bring to the boil, then simmer until completely soft. Mash with a fork and set aside to cool.

Into a large bowl, stir together the spelt flour, oats, raisins, baking powder, bicarbonate of/baking soda, cinnamon, mixed/apple pie spice, nutmeg and salt. Add the eggs, yogurt, mashed cooking apple, maple syrup and chopped eating apple. Combine together.

Spoon the mixture into it the prepared muffin pan. Bake in the preheated oven for about 30 minutes. A skewer should come out pretty much clean but a tiny bit of the muffin mixture on the skewer is OK, as it will continue to cook a little while cooling, leaving you with a nice moist middle.

For an after-dinner treat, you can serve the muffins with soy yogurt mixed with a little maple syrup and ground cinnamon.

Guilt-free because…

Pure maple syrup – high grade, 100% pure as opposed to 'maple-flavoured' sugar syrup – is great in baked goods. Recent research has discovered a number of compounds that may help fight cancer, infection and even type 1 diabetes. Five of these compounds have never been seen before and showed antioxidant and anti-inflammatory abilities. Phenols were also found in maple syrup to help toward the management of type 2 diabetes.

Stone fruit works brilliantly here, as once baked, their flavour and texture mellows out and their juices run down into the frangipane base, making for a deliciously moist and chewy tart. You can swap the nectarines for plums, peaches, cherries or pretty much any other stone fruit. I have included options for either healthy spelt flour or wheat- and gluten-free tart shell, and given how loaded with sugar, dairy and wheat a normal frangipane tart is, this is a minor miracle!

nectarine frangipane tart

Pastry
225 g/1¾ cups white spelt flour (for a wheat- and gluten-free alternative, see page 124)
pinch of sea salt
3 teaspoons xylitol
50 g/3 tablespoons dairy-free butter, e.g. sunflower spread
60 g/¼ cup hard white vegetable shortening (it is crucial that you get the hardest one you can find)
1 egg, beaten together with 1 teaspoon water

Frangipane Filling
70 g/½ cup pecans
80 g/⅔ cup blanched almonds
70 g/½ cup cashews
250 g/8¾ oz. dairy-free butter, e.g. sunflower or soy spread
40 g/3 tablespoons coconut oil
200 g/1 cup xylitol
grated zest of a lemon
3 eggs, lightly beaten
small handful of rice flour
pinch of sea salt
5 nectarines
sugar-free apricot jam, to glaze

20-cm/8-inch tart pan
baking beans

Serves 10

To make the pastry, follow the method for the Lemon Tart on page 124 until you have blind-baked the tart and taken it out to cool. Leave the oven on.

To make the frangipane filling, spread the pecans, almonds and cashews on a baking sheet and bake in the oven for about 8 minutes or until they have gone a shade darker. Allow to cool, then blitz in a food processor. You want to keep them a little chunky so don't grind them to a powder – about 10–15 seconds will probably do it. Set aside.

Put the butter, coconut oil, xylitol and lemon zest in the food processor. Blitz until light and fluffy. Remove to a large mixing bowl and beat in the eggs, rice flour, salt and, finally, the cooled nuts. Allow to cool and set in the fridge for at least 10 minutes.

When ready to bake, cut segments out of the nectarines. Spread the frangipane mixture over the blind-baked tart shell and arrange the nectarine segments on top in a fan pattern. Bake in the oven for about 45–55 minutes. The edges usually brown faster than the middle so I cover them with foil after about 25 minutes or when golden.

Remove the tart from the oven when the middle has browned and firmed up but is still a little wobbly when you gently shake it. Once cool, mix some of the apricot jam with a little hot water and, using a pastry brush, glaze the nectarines. Serve immediately.

Guilt-free because...

Nectarines are high in all the 'eye-health' nutrients, such as betacarotene (which the body converts into vitamin A), lutein, lycopene, zeaxanthin and beta-cryptoxanthin. These polyphenolic antioxidants have been shown in numerous trials to help prevent eye conditions such as cataracts and macular degeneration.

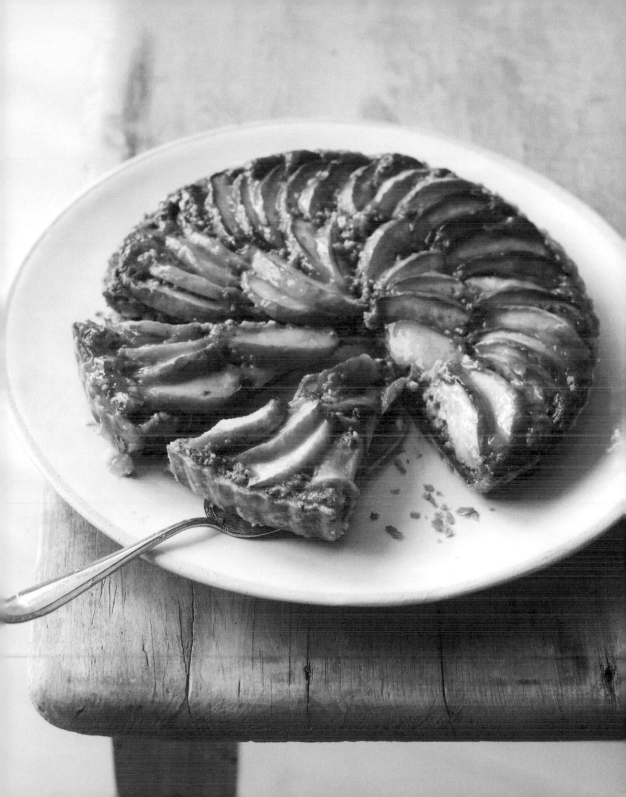

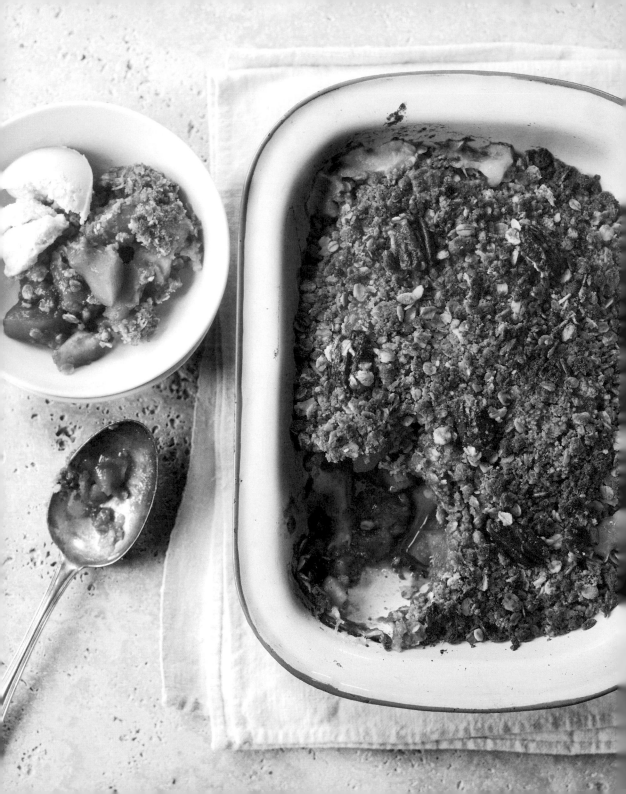

A few years ago I went back to Ireland for a job that went on all day and well into the night. It was the dead of winter and as the job required I be outside for a large portion of the day, I was frozen. Those of you who have experienced the particular brand of wet Irish winters will know exactly what I am talking about. I arrived home after 10 pm to the comforting smell of apple crumble, which my sister had made and was still warm sitting on the counter top. I ate an enormous portion with a big blob of ice cream. This is exactly what apple crumble is all about: warmth, familiarity and comfort.

pear & apple pecan crumble

Coconut Frozen Yogurt
   (page 135), to serve
   (optional)

Filling
2 cooking apples, eg.
   Lord Derby, Bramley,
   Pippin, Winesap
2 pears
80 g/scant ½ cup coconut
   palm sugar or 50 g/
   ¼ cup xylitol (coconut
   sugar is marginally
   better for this recipe)
juice of ½ lemon
60 g/½ cup pecans,
   lightly roasted

Topping
30 g/2 tablespoons
   sunflower spread
30 g/2 tablespoons
   coconut oil
70 g/½ cup plus
   1 tablespoon rice flour
70 g/½ cup rolled oats
60 g/⅓ cup coconut palm
   sugar or xylitol
2 tablespoons pure maple
   syrup
1 teaspoon ground
   cinnamon

medium pie dish or
   casserole dish

Serves 6–8

To make the filling, peel and core the apples and pears. Cut into large chunks and toss in a large saucepan with the coconut sugar, lemon juice and 1 tablespoon water. Stew over low–medium heat until half cooked. Taste and add more coconut sugar if necessary. Transfer to the pie dish or casserole dish with all the juices and mix in the pecans (reserving some for the top). Allow to cool while you make the topping.

Preheat the oven to 180°C (350°F) Gas 4.

To make the topping, in a large bowl, rub the sunflower spread and coconut oil into the flour until you have fine breadcrumbs. Add the oats, sugar, maple syrup and cinnamon and mix thoroughly. Sprinkle the topping over the filling in the dish and bake in the preheated oven for about 35–45 minutes or until the fruit is tender and the juices bubbling. Sprinkle the remaining pecans over the top and serve with a blob of Coconut Frozen Yogurt, if you like.

Guilt-free because…

Apples certainly live up to their saying: 'an apple a day keeps the doctor away'. The phyto-nutrients found in apples, such as quercetin, kaempferol, myricetin and chlorogenic acid act as antioxidants within the body and have been researched for their potential role in cardiovascular health, blood sugar regulation and their anti-asthma and anti-cancer benefits. Apple consumption has been found to be most beneficial for colon, breast and lung cancers, so it's an invaluable addition to any diet.

On the way home from school as a teenager I used to love stopping off at a little bake shop run by a hilarious team of old ladies, to buy some of their homemade flapjacks. They were almost intoxicatingly buttery and syrupy… delicious, but it somehow managed to defeat the purpose of the healthy oats, by drowning them in all that sugar. After tricking around with a few different ingredients, my sister and I came up with these flapjacks, which are just as delicious and chewy, and dare I say it, intoxicating, while still being good for you.

flapjacks

100 g/6½ tablespoons coconut oil
20 g/4 teaspoons sunflower spread
130 ml/½ cup sunflower oil
2 ripe bananas, mashed
2 teaspoons pure vanilla extract
140 g/¾ cup xylitol or coconut palm sugar
60 ml/¼ cup agave syrup
1 tablespoon date syrup
good pinch of sea salt
500 g/4 cups rolled oats
150 g/1 cup raisins
100 g/¾ cup pumpkin seeds
60 g/½ cup pecans
100 g/⅔ cup unsulphured dried apricots, chopped

baking pan, about 20–25 cm/ 8–10 inches

Serves 10–12

Preheat the oven to 180˚C (350˚F) Gas 4.

Gently heat the coconut oil, margarine, sunflower oil, bananas, vanilla extract, xylitol or coconut sugar, agave syrup, date syrup and salt in a saucepan just until the margarine has melted. Whisk the mixture together until smooth.

In a large mixing bowl, combine the oats, raisins, pumpkin seeds, pecans and apricots. Add the molten mixture from the pan and mix very well. Spoon the mixture into the baking pan and flatten down tightly to help it hold together. Bake in the preheated oven for about 25 minutes or until the flapjacks are a lovely golden, light brown colour. If it looks like they are colouring too quickly, turn the heat down to 160˚C (325˚F) Gas 3. The main thing is not to burn the top, as the raisins and apricots burn easily and become very bitter.

With flapjacks, you really can make them your own. If you are less keen on the dried fruit, take it out or add other nuts or seeds. The choice is yours.

Guilt-free because…

Oats are a great source of soluble fibre. A part of this fibre called beta-glucan is effective at lowering blood cholesterol, as it 'traps' some of the substances relating to cholesterol absorption, thereby reducing the amount of cholesterol that may enter the bloodstream. Harvard School of Public Health have conducted studies showing that eating oats may lead to improved metabolic health, thereby reducing the chances of long-term weight gain. Use organic oats if you can. Oats are naturally gluten free but many brands process them in factories that process wheat. Oats processed in wheat-free factories should be labelled 'gluten-free'.

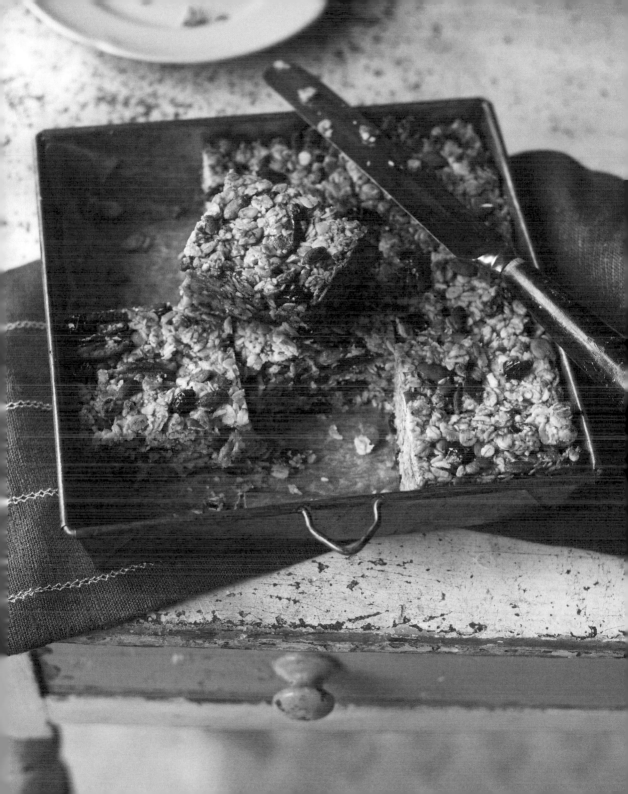

orange-zest brownies

225 g/7½ oz. dark/ bittersweet chocolate, at least 70% cocoa solids (there is a very minimal amount of sugar in the ingredients of dark/bittersweet chocolate. If you want no sugar at all you can buy sugar-free dark/ bittersweet chocolate in health stores), chopped

110 g/1 cup rice flour

70 g/½ cup plus 1 tablespoon unsweetened cocoa powder

½ teaspoon baking powder

½ teaspoon sea salt

225 g/7 oz. dairy-free butter, e.g. sunflower or soy spread

170 g/¾ cup coconut palm sugar or xylitol

2 eggs

2 egg yolks

grated zest of 1 orange

100 g/⅔ cup pecans, lightly roasted

small baking pan or roasting pan, lined with parchment paper

Serves 10–12

Guilt-free because...

Xylitol is natural sugar alcohol that is a great alternative to processed sugar. It helps prevent tooth decay because the mouth bacteria can't convert it into damaging acids that attack tooth enamel. In small amounts, it also helps decrease the formation of plaque.

Preheat the oven to 180°C (350°F) Gas 4.

Melt the chocolate in a heatproof bowl over a saucepan of simmering water, making sure the base of the bowl does not touch the water.

Sift the flour, cocoa powder, baking powder and salt into a bowl. In another bowl, beat the butter with the sugar until pale and fluffy. Slowly mix in the eggs and egg yolks, then the melted chocolate and orange zest. Finally, stir in the sifted ingredients and pecans. As the melted chocolate cools, the mixture becomes increasingly stiff and difficult to mix, to the point that you may think you have made a mistake and need to add more liquid... but don't! This is what makes these brownies so decadently chewy and dense in texture. If you have a food mixer it makes the job a little easier, otherwise work those triceps!

Spoon the mixture into the prepared baking pan and, with the back of a metal spoon, level the top. Dipping the spoon into hot water every now and again prevents it from sticking. Bake in the preheated oven for about 20 minutes, depending on your oven and the thickness of your brownie. It should be slightly undercooked and a skewer should come out with some of the wet mixture still on it, as the brownie will firm up once it has cooled and the chocolate sets. Once cool, transfer to the fridge until fully set, then cut into small squares and devour!

Honestly, who doesn't love a good sticky and chewy chocolate brownie? They are the ultimate in decadent home baking – rich and moist and totally addictive. This recipe is completely sin free, yet still delicious and indulgent-tasting. I have had people beg me for the recipe when they found out they were sugar, wheat and dairy free.

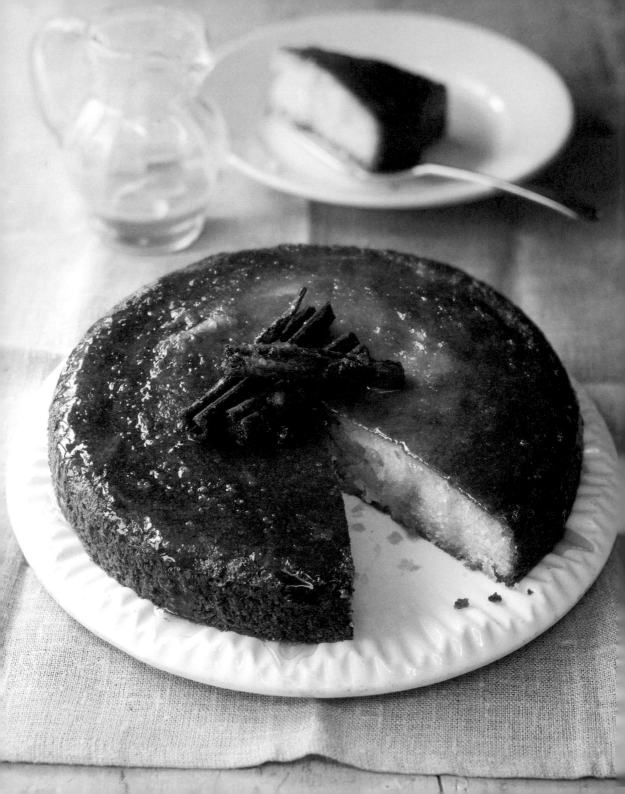

Naturally wheat free (it is made with ground almonds) and supremely moist, drowned in a sweet orange syrup, this exotic cake never fails to impress. My mother used to buy a cake similar to this as a special treat for the family. Without fail the time would come when someone could be heard hollering: 'who finished the cake? There was half left this morning!' Something akin to the Spanish Inquisition would then follow, but mysteriously the culprit would never be found. Naturally, I had absolutely nothing to do with it.

moroccan orange cake

300 g/1½ cups ground almonds
250 g/1⅓ cups xylitol
2 teaspoons baking powder
5 eggs
200 ml/¾ cup plus 1 tablespoon sunflower oil
2 teaspoons agave syrup for the cake, plus 60 ml/5 tablespoons for the syrup
grated zest and juice of 1 large orange
grated zest and juice of ½ lemon
3 cloves
3 cinnamon sticks
soy yogurt with some ground cinnamon stirred though, to serve

20-cm/8-inch springform pan, baselined with parchment paper

Serves 10–12

Preheat the oven to 180˚C (350˚F) Gas 4.

In a bowl, mix together the ground almonds, xylitol and baking powder. In a separate bowl, whisk together the eggs, sunflower oil, the 2 teaspoons of agave syrup and the orange and lemon zest. Pour the mixture into the dry ingredients and combine together.

Pour the cake mixture into the prepared baking pan and bake in the preheated oven for 35–45 minutes until a skewer inserted in the middle comes out clean. If the top looks like it is going to burn, cover with foil, being careful not to press on the cake. Allow to cool slightly while you make a syrup.

Put the orange and lemon juices, the 60 ml/5 tablespoons agave syrup, cloves and cinnamon in a saucepan. Bring to the boil, reduce the heat and simmer for 5 minutes.

While the cake is still warm, turn it out onto a plate, drizzle the syrup over and allow it to seep in. If it is not all absorbed at once, keep it aside to drizzle over later. When you are ready to serve, pile the cinnamon sticks and cloves on top of one another on the cake. Serve with the cinnamon-soy yogurt dolloped onto each slice.

Making a tart free of sugar, wheat and dairy that tastes as good as the normal one seemed almost impossible at first but I got there in the end. I have included a spelt-flour version for the tart shell, which although not entirely wheat free, still has far less gluten and is much better for you than regular flour.

lemon tart

Pastry

225 g/1¾ cups white spelt flour or gluten-free flour blend, or to make your own, combine 100 g/¾ cup rice flour, 70 g/¾ cup cornflour/cornstarch, 55 g/½ cup potato flour and 1 teaspoon xanthan gum

pinch of sea salt

1 dessertspoon xylitol

50 g/3 tablespoons dairy-free butter, e.g. sunflower spread

60 g/¼ cup hard white vegetable shortening (it is crucial that you get the hardest one you can find)

1 egg, beaten together with 1 teaspoon water

Filling

finely grated zest and juice of 3 lemons

juice of 1 orange

120 g/⅔ cup xylitol

4 eggs

160 ml/⅔ cup soy cream/creamer

soy yogurt and raspberries, to serve

20-cm/8-inch tart pan

baking beans

Serves 10–12

The pastry ingredients must be as cold as possible, especially the butter and shortening, so refrigerate until needed.

Sift the flour (and xanthan gum if you are making the gluten-free version) and salt into a large bowl. Add the xylitol, butter and shortening and cut into small chunks with a knife. With your hands high, rub the butter and shortening into the flour until it resembles breadcrumbs. You can also do this in a food processor. Add a tablespoon of the egg mixture and fork the mixture together. If it is still crumbly and not coming together, add a little more liquid, being careful not to overdo it. Bring the dough together with your hands to a smooth ball, with no crumbs falling away. For the gluten-free version, you will need to squeeze and knead the pastry a little. If it is still crumbly, it needs a little more egg mixture. Gently flatten into a round, wrap in clingfilm/plastic wrap and refrigerate until cold.

Preheat the oven to 180°C (350°F) Gas 4.

Gluten-free pastry is quite difficult to handle, as there is no gluten to help bind everything together, so I roll it out between 2 sheets of floured clingfilm/plastic wrap. Whichever pastry you have made, roll it out until 1 cm/⅜ inch thick, working quickly and handling it as little as possible. To line the tart pan, remove the top layer of film/wrap and roll the pastry over your rolling pin with the bottom sheet of film/wrap still on it. Lay the sheet of pastry over the pan with the film/wrap now uppermost. Remove the film/wrap.

The gluten-free pastry will tear and crumble as you transfer it to the pan but this is quite normal, and although it looks like a shambles now it will be fine once blindbaked. Patch it up with the pieces that have fallen off and push the pastry into the pan, making sure there is an even thickness and there are no cracks. Prick the base with a fork. Line the pastry shell with parchment paper and fill with baking beans.

Blind-bake in the preheated oven for about 20 minutes. (Leave the oven on.) Remove the paper and beans and brush the base and sides of the shell with egg mixture. Return to the oven and bake for a further 5–10 minutes until the base is beginning to brown. Remove and cool on a wire rack.

To make the filling, whisk the citrus zest, juices and xylitol in a pan and gently heat until the xylitol has just dissolved. Allow to cool, then whisk in the eggs and soy cream/creamer. Place the tart shell in the oven, then pour the filling in, right up to the top. Bake until the filling is just firm and doesn't wobble too much when the tart is moved from side to side – about 20 minutes. Serve with soy yogurt and raspberries.

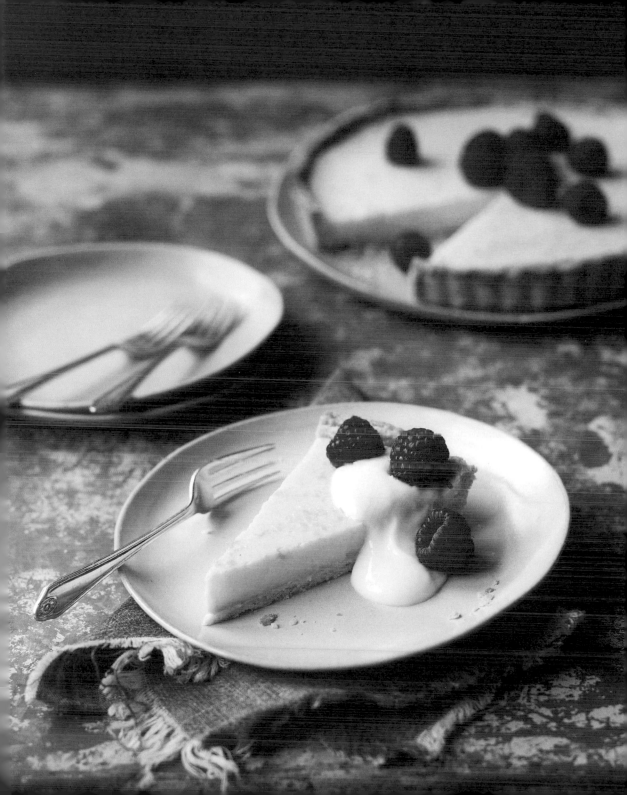

sweet treats

From truffles and ice cream to chocolate tart and cheesecake, this chapter shows you how to be indulgent the good-for-you way! So go on, give in to temptation and enjoy these decadent yet guilt-free sweet treats!

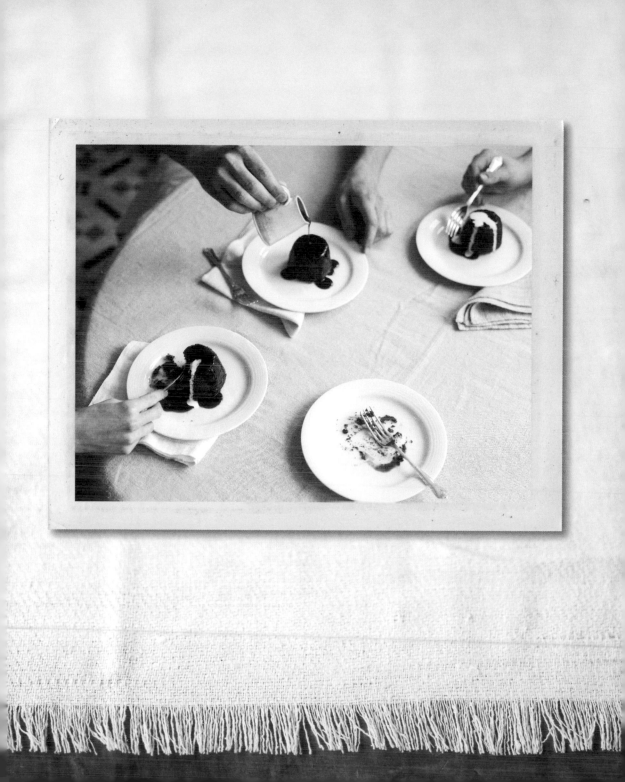

Convincing people that food, especially desserts, made without sugar, wheat and dairy can actually taste good, let alone delicious, is an almost impossible task, which is why I adore this chocolate tart. It will convert even the greatest cynics who protest that no dessert free of sugar, wheat and dairy could possibly taste as good as their more sinful cousins. After tasting this, I guarantee your family and friends will admit defeat and beg you for the recipe, as well as another slice!

chocolate tart

sea salt
100 g/3½ oz. best-quality dark/bittersweet chocolate, at least 70% cocoa solids

Base
10 pitted dates
150 g/1 cup pecans, lightly roasted
125 g/4 oz. Scottish oat cakes
1 teaspoon pure vanilla extract
2 tablespoons agave syrup
2 tablespoons coconut oil
3 teaspoons unsweetened cocoa powder

Filling
3 avocados, not too firm
4 tablespoons coconut oil
6 tablespoons agave syrup
1 tablespoon carob powder
5 tablespoons unsweetened cocoa powder
2 teaspoons pure vanilla extract
3 tablespoons date syrup

20-cm/8-inch springform pan, baselined with parchment paper

Serves 10–12

To make the base, blitz the dates in a food processor, then add the rest of the ingredients and a pinch of salt and blitz until everything comes together into a sticky ball.

Press into the baking pan so that you have an even and smooth base for the tart. Refrigerate for 30 minutes or freeze for 15 minutes until set.

To make the filling, cut the avocados in half, remove the stones and scoop the flesh into a food processor. Add ½ teaspoon salt, the remaining ingredients apart from the coconut oil, and blitz until smooth.

Melt the coconut oil in a pan over the lowest heat possible – this will only take a few moments. Turn on the food processor and pour the coconut oil into the mixture through the funnel. Once combined, pour the mixture onto the set tart base and smooth out the top. Refrigerate for at least 2 hours or if you want it to set quickly, freeze it.

When you are ready to serve, warm the chocolate to just above room temperature to make it easier to grate. I find leaving it beside the oven when you are cooking for about 10 minutes does the trick. You want the chocolate to be just beginning to soften – not in any way gooey or melting, just not rock solid, so it grates easily in long strips.

Pop the tart out of the baking pan and transfer to a plate. Liberally grate the chocolate over, so it piles up high. The tart should be served fridge-cold so that it stays reasonably firm. It keeps wonderfully well and can easily be made a day in advance.

Guilt-free because…

Avocados are high in essential omega fats, which are food for the brain, nervous system, skin and hair. Contrary to popular belief, avocados do not make you fat! In fact, studies have shown that those who have high amounts of healthy fats like avocados (and indeed coconut oil) in their diet are more likely to be a healthy weight.

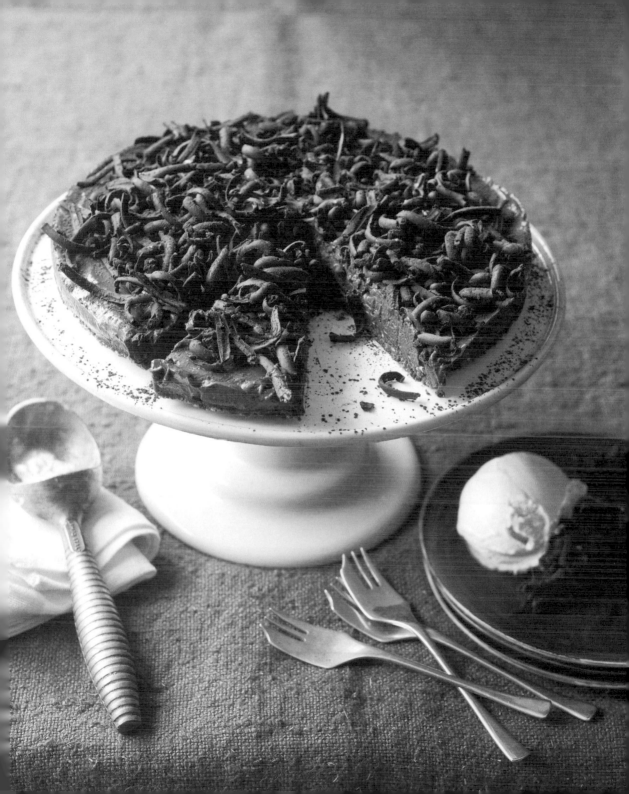

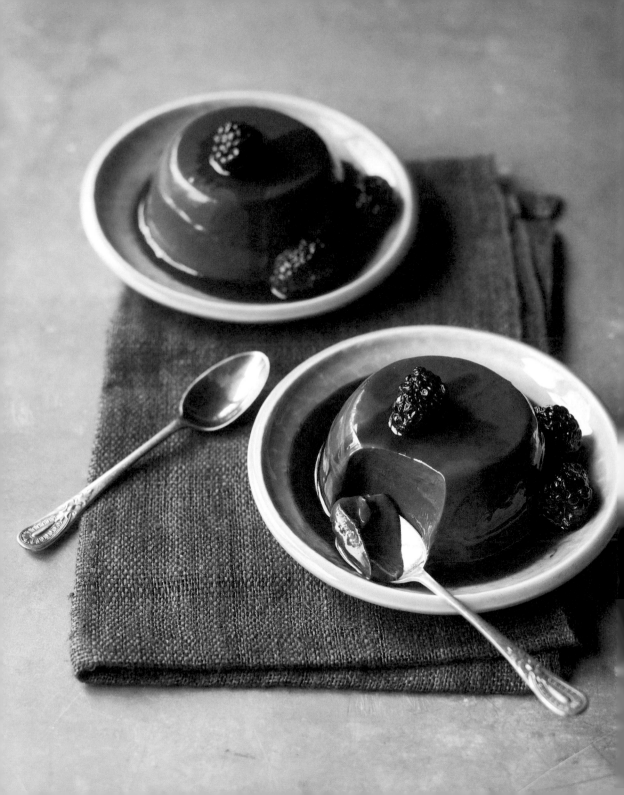

Skye Gyngell, the Michelin-starred chef with whom I trained at Petersham Nurseries restaurant and whose knowledge and innate understanding of food I am in constant awe of, explained how the chocolate works marvellously well in this panna cotta, blending seamlessly into the mixture and making for a really rich and creamy dessert. I adapted Skye's recipe for a client who was off dairy and sugar and it was a resounding success.

skye gyngell's chocolate panna cotta

5 half or 2 full sheets leaf gelatine (if you are vegetarian, use agar flakes and follow the packet instructions, as you will require less agar than gelatine)
200 g/6½ oz. best-quality dark/bittersweet chocolate, at least 70% cocoa solids, chopped
190 ml/¾ cup rice milk
250 ml/1 cup soy cream/creamer
90 g/½ cup xylitol
1 vanilla bean, split lengthways
handful of blackberries warmed with a little agave syrup, to serve (optional)

4 dariole moulds or ramekins

Serves 4

Lightly oil the moulds with vegetable oil (but do not oil them if you are using agar flakes, as the oil prevents the agar from setting).

Soak the gelatine leaves in water to soften them.

Melt the chocolate in a heatproof bowl over a saucepan of simmering water, making sure the base of the bowl does not touch the water.

While the chocolate is melting, put the milk, soy cream/creamer, xylitol and vanilla bean and its seeds, scraped out, into a heavy-based pan and bring to a gentle simmer, stirring occasionally until the xylitol has dissolved. Remove from the heat and strain through a sieve/strainer into the melted chocolate, mixing as you pour, until well mixed.

Squeeze the excess water out of the gelatine leaves and add to the chocolate mixture, stirring to dissolve. Strain through a sieve/strainer into a jug or measuring cup and use this to pour the mixture into the moulds. Allow to cool, then refrigerate for at least 2 hours or until set.

To serve, dip the moulds into boiling water for a couple of seconds to loosen the sides. Place a plate on top and then flip over; you may need to shake the panna cotta to release it from the mould.

Skye serves this with blackberries, which she warms up in a pan with some honey. It is a wonderful combination that also works well with agave syrup or maple syrup.

Guilt-free because…

Dark/bittersweet chocolate, unlike its 'milkier' counterpart, is high in antioxidants, which help reduce the 'bad' LDL cholesterol. It also has flavonoids, which maintain blood pressure and reduce the chance of blood clots. Opt for high-quality chocolate with a minimum cocoa content of 70% – ideally 80% – for optimal health benefits with minimal sugar consumption.

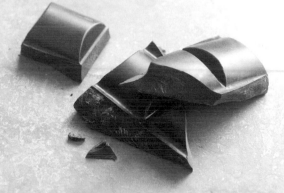

I scream, you scream, we all scream for ice cream! One of life's greatest pleasures has to be the cool, sweet, creamy smoothness of homemade ice cream. This is one of those recipes, a bit like the chocolate tart on page 128, that people simply cannot get their heads around. The notion that something this creamy and indulgent could actually be free of sugar and dairy and still taste this good, is just beyond them.

cashew butter ice cream

180 g/1 cup xylitol
6 egg yolks
400 ml/1⅔ cups rice milk
400 ml/1⅔ cups soy cream/creamer
1 vanilla bean, split lengthways
200 g/1 scant cup cashew butter (available in supermarkets and health food stores)
3 tablespoons agave syrup

ice cream machine (optional)

Serves 6

For any ice cream, you start with a crème anglaise. Once you have this base, you can experiment with whatever ingredients you love: stewed fruit or melted chocolate (for stracciatella) are my favourites, but nuts or herbs are also good – in fact the possibilities are endless!

Put the xylitol and egg yolks in a bowl (or stand mixer) and, using an electric whisk, whisk until light and fluffy and pale yellow in colour.

Put the milk, soy cream/creamer and vanilla bean in a heavy-based saucepan and bring to the boil. After a minute, turn off the heat and allow to cool slightly.

Add the warm cream mixture to the egg mixture, whisking constantly and vigorously to prevent the egg from curdling. When it is all combined, pour the mixture back into the saucepan and place over low heat. Using a plastic spatula, stir the mixture constantly in a figure-eight motion. After about 5–10 minutes the

mixture will have thickened and will coat the back of a wooden spoon – drag your finger across the back of the spoon and if the line holds and does not drip, you have got the right consistency. Be careful though, as it can turn into scrambled eggs very easily if the heat is too high.

If you have an ice cream machine, use this to churn the mixture according to the manufacturer's instructions.

If you don't have an ice cream machine, pour the mixture into a freezerproof container (wide, flat, metal trays work well as the mixture freezes more quickly) and freeze.

After 30 minutes, or when the edges are beginning to freeze, remove the container from the freezer and whisk thoroughly to break down the ice crystals. Repeat this process twice more at 30-minute intervals. At this point, mix together the cashew butter and agave syrup and stir through the ice cream, so you have lovely cashew streaks and swirls, then return to the freezer to set fully.

Remove from the freezer about 15 minutes before serving so that it softens up a little – you want it smooth and creamy.

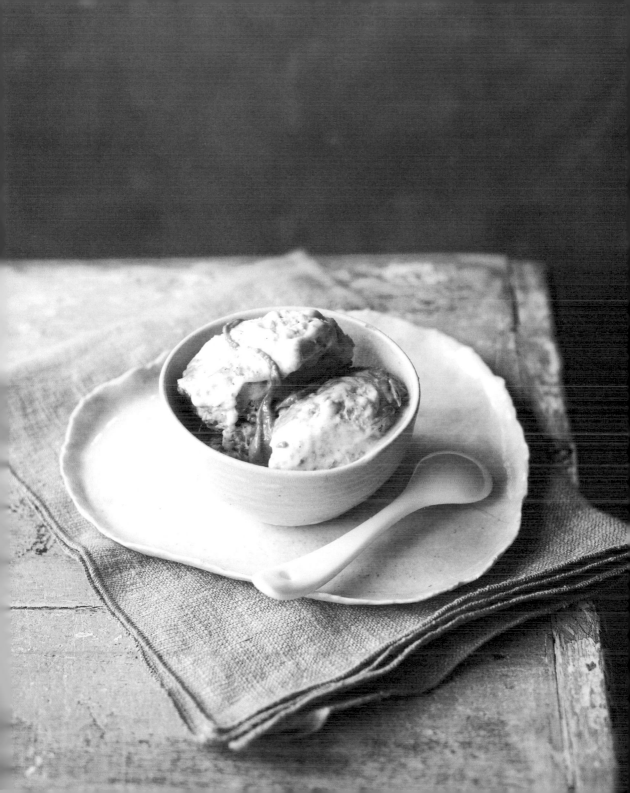

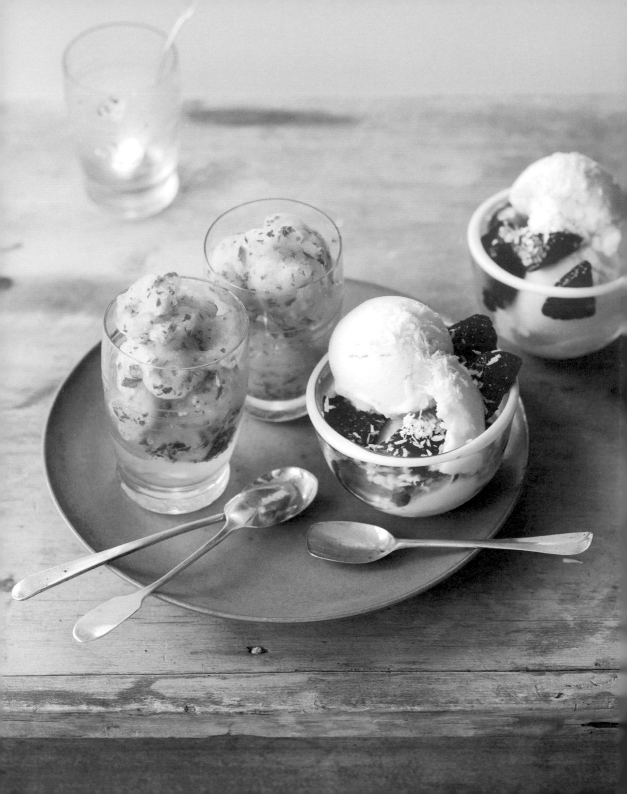

Frozen yogurt is going through a bit of a renaissance at the moment and it's not hard to see why. Fresh and light with only a fraction of the fat of ice cream, it is the natural choice for the health conscious. It is still made with dairy though, so I came up with this recipe using soy yogurt and coconut milk. All you need is a freezer!

A few years ago, I was planning a menu for a dinner party when it occurred to me that the mojito I had been drinking the previous night might also make a great sorbet. I came up with this recipe and thankfully it went down a storm. You also have the added value of being able to use any leftover sorbet to make a killer mojito smoothie!

coconut frozen yogurt
with strawberries

700 ml/1 lb. 8 oz. plain soy yogurt
340 ml/1½ cups coconut milk
100 ml/⅓ cup plus 1 tablespoon agave syrup
2 teaspoons lemon juice

desiccated coconut, to serve
strawberries, to serve

ice cream machine (optional)

Serves 6–8

Put the yogurt, milk, agave syrup and lemon juice in a bowl and mix until smooth. If you have an ice cream machine, use this to churn the mixture according to the manufacturer's instructions.

If you don't have an ice cream machine, pour the mixture into a freezerproof container (wide, flat, metal trays work well as the mixture freezes more quickly) and freeze. After 30 minutes, or when the edges are beginning to freeze, remove the container from the freezer and whisk thoroughly to break down the ice crystals. Return to the freezer and repeat this process intermittently until completely frozen, but do not let it go rock hard, as you want to be able to scoop it out easily. If you want it super smooth, you can blitz it in a food processor when it is just frozen.

Scoop into a bowl and serve with strawberries and desiccated coconut over the top.

The variations for this are endless. For a plain version, use rice milk instead of coconut milk. Add any blitzed up fruit or cocoa powder. Play around with it!

mojito sorbet

170 g/1 cup xylitol
5 sprigs of fresh mint plus 2 tablespoons freshly chopped leaves

grated zest and juice of 2 limes

ice cream machine (optional)

Serves 6–8

Put 500 ml/2 cups water, the xylitol and mint sprigs in a saucepan and bring to the boil. Reduce the heat to a minimum and simmer for 5 minutes.

Remove from the heat and strain the liquid, squeezing as much liquid as possible out of the sprigs. Immediately, while the liquid is still hot, add the lime zest. Allow the mixture to cool slightly, then add the lime juice and chopped mint leaves. Refrigerate to cool thoroughly.

If you have an ice cream machine, use this to churn the mixture according to the manufacturer's instructions.

If you don't have an ice cream machine, pour the mixture into a freezerproof container (wide, flat, metal trays work well as the mixture freezes more quickly) and freeze. After 20 minutes, or when the edges are beginning to freeze, remove the container from the freezer and whisk thoroughly to break down the ice crystals. This will ensure a smooth sorbet. Return to the freezer and repeat this process intermittently until the sorbet is frozen.

Chocolate truffles are the ultimate in stolen, sinful pleasures. I think their size may have something to do with it, as in one fell swoop you can have that ball of chocolatey goodness devoured and no one is any the wiser. This is a recipe for the most indulgent, yet guilt-free truffles you will ever taste, using a few healthy alternatives. This may seem like a contradiction, but just taste one and you will understand.

chocolate truffles

handful of pecans and
    hazelnuts
sea salt
150 ml/⅔ cup soy
    cream/creamer
30 g/2 tablespoons
    coconut oil
200 g/6½ oz. dark/
    bittersweet chocolate,
    at least 70% cocoa
    solids: 150 g/5 oz. of it
    grated, and the rest
    chopped (You can also
    use sugar-free dark/
    bittersweet chocolate)
1 tablespoon xylitol or
    coconut palm sugar
grated zest of ½ orange
unsweetened cocoa
    powder
1 teaspoon sunflower oil

2 skewers

Makes 24–28

Preheat the oven to 180°C (350°F) Gas 4.

Roast the nuts on a baking sheet in the preheated oven for 10 minutes or until they have gone a shade darker. Allow to cool, then crush or finely chop with a pinch of salt.

Put the soy cream/creamer and coconut oil in a saucepan until hot and the coconut oil has melted but is not simmering. Add the grated chocolate, xylitol and a pinch of salt while stirring quickly with a whisk. Keep whisking until all the chocolate has melted and you have a smooth mixture. Transfer to a bowl, keeping a third aside. Mix this third with the orange zest. Allow them all to cool, then cover with clingfilm/plastic wrap and refrigerate for at least 4 hours or until more solid and pliable.

To shape the truffles, keep the mixture in the fridge if you can and try to handle it as little as possible, as the warmth of your hands will melt it. I run my hands under cold water for as long as I can bare it to begin with. Dry your hands, then coat them in cocoa powder. Take a teaspoon of the mixture and quickly roll it between flat hands until you have a neat ball shape, then place on a plate in the fridge. Continue until you have made all the mixture into little truffles, doing the

same with the orange-zest mixture. Refrigerate for at least 1 hour or until fully cool.

To make chocolate-coated truffles, melt the chopped chocolate and sunflower oil in a heatproof bowl over a saucepan of simmering water, making sure the base of the bowl does not touch the water. Insert a skewer about 1 cm/½ inch into the base of one of the truffles, then dip it into the melted chocolate, quickly swirling it around to make sure it is completely covered. Using a second skewer, slide the truffle off the tip and onto a plate lined with parchment paper. Continue until you have coated half of the plain truffles. Once the chocolate has set, put the plate in the fridge until ready to serve.

Roll the remaining plain truffles between warm hands to soften the outside slightly, then roll in the nuts until completely covered and place in the fridge. Roll the orange-zest truffles in cocoa powder and shake off any excess. Refrigerate with the others.

Remove the truffles from the fridge about 10 minutes before you want to serve them. You can place them in little paper truffle cases or pile them into a little bag as a gift. They keep well in the fridge but are best enjoyed as soon as possible, which won't be a problem!

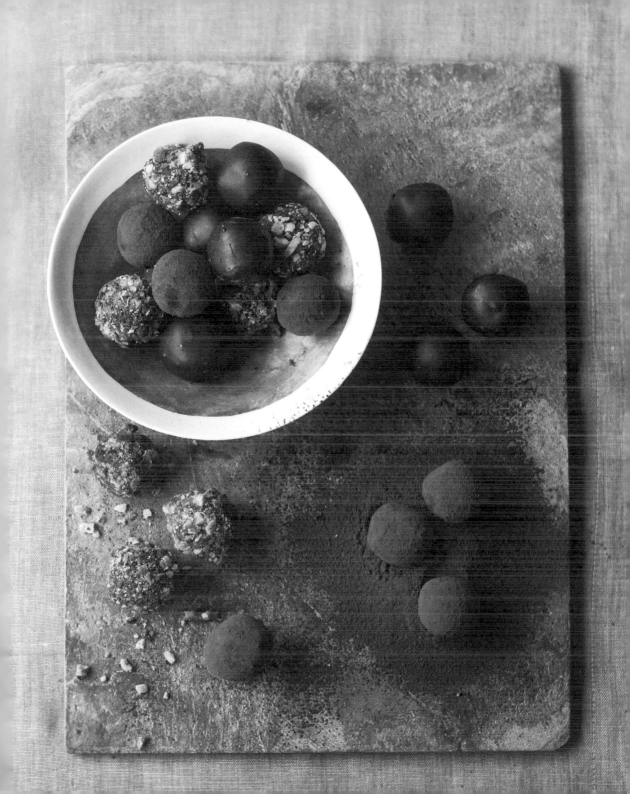

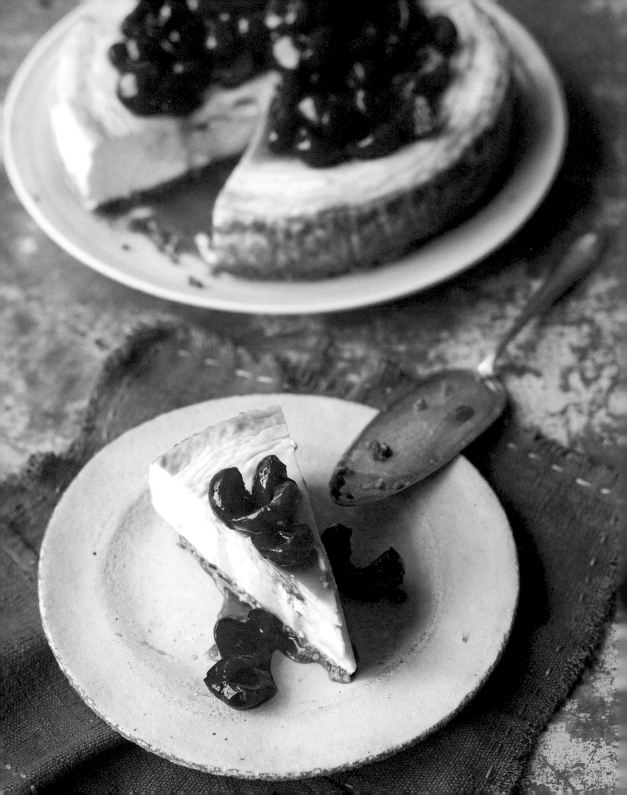

Achieving that cloying, deeply creamy goodness of a cheesecake without dairy was long a mission of mine. There are a number of ways you can get excellent results using cashews or silken tofu, but for a cheesecake that no one will know is dairy free, I find the 'Tofutti' brand of dairy-free cream cheese is the answer. Made from soy and non-hydrogenated vegetable oils, it is identical to normal cream cheese in taste and texture, especially in this glorious dessert.

cheesecake & sweet cherries

500 g/1 lb. fresh cherries, pitted
4 tablespoons agave syrup

Base
150 g/1 cup pecans
150 g/5 oz. Scottish oatcakes
80 g/5½ tablespoons coconut oil
2 tablespoons agave syrup
good pinch of sea salt

Filling
900 g/1 lb. 14 oz. Tofutti Cream Cheese
grated zest of 5 lemons and juice of 1
130 g/¾ cup xylitol
5 eggs
1 tablespoon rice flour
2 teaspoons pure vanilla extract
pinch of sea salt

20-cm/8-inch springform pan, lined with baking parchment

Serves 10–12

Preheat the oven to 180°C (350°F) Gas 4.

To make the base, roast the pecans on a baking sheet in the preheated oven for 10 minutes or until they have gone a shade darker. Allow to cool slightly and leave the oven on.

Melt the coconut oil in a pan over the lowest heat possible – this will only take a few moments. Crush the oatcakes and roasted pecans in a food processor or in a sealed bag with a rolling pin, then transfer to a bowl with the melted coconut oil, agave syrup and salt and mix very well. Press into the baking pan so that you have an even and smooth base for the cheesecake.

To make the filling, put all the ingredients in a food processor and blitz until well combined. Pour the mixture onto the set cheesecake base and smooth out the top. Bake for about 45 minutes or until it is just set and the middle is still a little wobbly. It will set further as it cools. Once completely cold, pop the cheesecake out of the baking pan and peel off the paper.

To serve, squash the cherries a little between your hands to release some of the juices. Add the agave syrup and mix together. Just before serving, pour onto the middle of the cheesecake and serve big wedges with the cherry liquid seeping down the sides.

Guilt-free because...

Cherries have garnered significant interest in recent years from those suffering with gout, due to their anti-inflammatory effect. Studies have shown that the particular polyphenol compound hat cherries contain (anthocyanins), blocks the actions of cyclooxygenase-1 and -2 enzymes, thus reducing the pain caused by inflammation. It has also been noted that athletes recover better after training and experience less muscle pain when consuming cherry juice before and after exercise. Cherries are extremely high in antioxidants, most notably melatonin. Melatonin can cross the blood-brain barrier, leading to a calming effect on brain neurons, which in turn may help those suffering with insomnia or nervous conditions.

Pudding

225 g/7½ oz. dates, pitted and chopped
200 ml/1 scant cup boiling water
100 ml/6 tablespoons rice milk
90 g/6 tablespoons dairy-free butter, e.g. sunflower spread
150 g/¾ cup coconut palm sugar
3 eggs
2 tablespoons date syrup
180 g/1½ cups gluten-free flour blend or rice flour
1 teaspoon baking powder
1 teaspoon bicarbonate of/baking soda
1 teaspoon pure vanilla extract
pinch of sea salt

Toffee Sauce

100 g/3½ oz. dairy-free butter, e.g. sunflower spread
175 g/¾ cup coconut palm sugar
1 tablespoon blackstrap molasses
100 ml/6 tablespoons maple syrup
½ teaspoon pure vanilla extract
230 ml/1 cup soy cream/creamer, plus extra to serve
pinch of sea salt

6–8 dariole moulds, depending on the size

Makes 6–8

I adore this traditional British dessert, but there is no denying that it really is not fantastic for you. I eventually figured out a way to achieve that deep, toffee taste without all the bad stuff to make this healthier version which is still wickedly good.

sticky toffee pudding

Preheat the oven to 180°C (350°F) Gas 4. Grease and flour the moulds, then line the bases with a disc of oiled parchment paper so that the puddings turn out more easily.

To make the pudding, soak the dates in the boiling water for 5 minutes, then blitz in a food processor until smooth. Add the remaining ingredients and blitz again until well combined. Spoon into the prepared moulds but not right to the top, as they rise quite a bit. Bake in the preheated oven for 20 minutes or until they are risen and firm. You can check the middle with a skewer. 10 minutes before they are

finished, make the toffee sauce. Melt the butter, sugar, molasses and maple syrup in a saucepan over low heat, then simmer for a few minutes. Gradually stir in the vanilla extract, soy cream/creamer and salt and bring to the boil for 1–2 minutes until slightly thickened.

Leave the puddings in their moulds for about 5 minutes, then turn onto plates and spoon the toffee sauce over and around with a little extra soy cream/creamer to top it off.

Say it with me: 'heaven!' You can also serve this with the Coconut Frozen Yogurt from page 135.

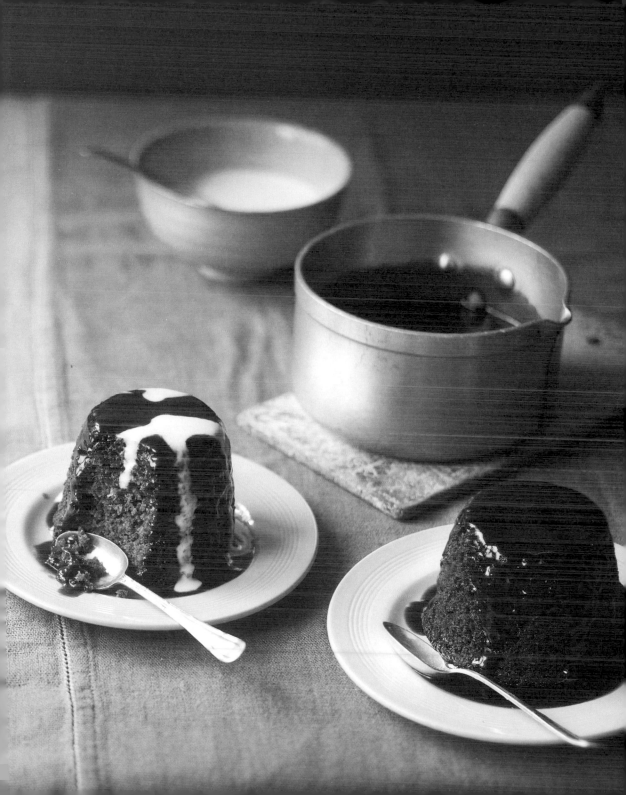

index

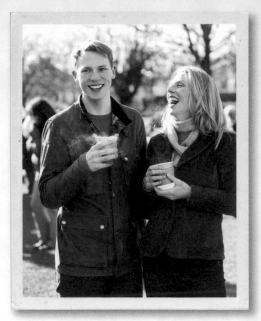

acknowledgments

To our family for their constant support, constructive criticism and encouragement; this book never would have happened without you all. Particularly, Jina and Jesse our respective spouses, for putting up with our non-stop Skype chats about food, food, food! And let's not forget Jessica's gorgeous children Rosa and Isaac, for being Mummy's little helpers in the kitchen!

A huge thank you to the whole team at Ryland Peters & Small for making this cookbook happen. Cindy for giving the book the go-ahead, Julia, Céline, and Leslie for shaping the book into its beautiful finished state, Liz for the fantastic props, Lauren for her PR prowess, and to Megan and Kate (and her dog Badger) who designed and photographed the book and were an absolute hoot to work with! Thank you also to my great cooking assistants Rosie, Fiona and Rhiannon and to Helen Ennis at Dunbeacon Pottery for the kind loan of her stunning crockery. Dunbeacon Pottery, Durrus, West Cork, Ireland. Telephone +353(0)27 61036 www.dunbeaconpottery.com.

To Skye Gyngell and all the wonderful chefs that I have worked with at Petersham Nurseries over the past two years, with whom I have learned so much about the importance of excellent-quality produce and simple, loving cooking, a big thank you. And to Darina, Rachel, Rory and the rest of the teachers at Ballymaloe, where it all began.

Finally, to our grandmother, the original cook in our family, for inspiring our love for food and gifting us her 1961 first edition copy of 'Larousse Gastronomique'.

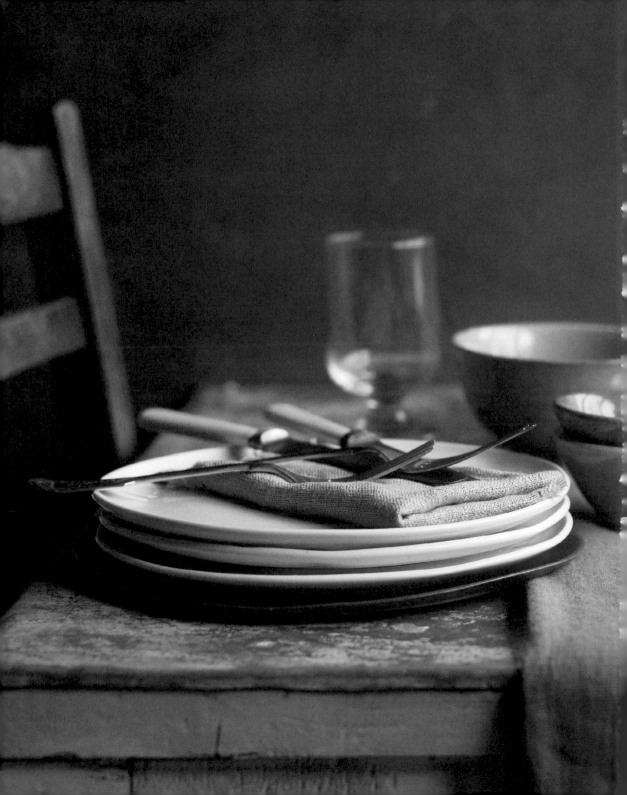